"Debbie Danowski is absolutely compassionate about how mired most of us are in false thoughts and images about ourselves and others. Her new book is brave, daring, funny, wise, and very inspiring. It is a must read for all of us."

—Jayne Atkinson, actress

"Once again, Dr. Danowski states some simple truths which, if followed, can not only change a person's eating habits but one's life. This book could easily be used in conjunction with therapy as a daily reinforcement of mentally healthy approaches to eating."

—Jocelyn Novella, LPC, NCC,
Creator of the Eating Disorders Task Force at Sacred Heart University

"This wonderful book is a gift as well as a tool in our arsenal against emotional eating—it is written with compassion and love. Keep this book close and read it when you feel lost and alone. It will inspire you."

—Tina A. compulsive overeater

Debbie Danowski, PhD, is a nationally renowned expert on weight loss. A pioneer in the food addictions field, she is the author of *Why Can't I Stop Eating?*, *Locked Up For Eating Too Much*, and *The Overeater's Journal*. For over twenty years, she has worked as a freelance writer, her articles appearing in *First for Women*, *Woman's Day*, and *Seventeen*, among other publications. She is on the International Advisory Board for the Food Addiction Institute and currently holds an associate professorship at Sacred Heart University in Fairfield, Connecticut. Visit her online at www.debbiedanowski.com.

THE
EMOTIONAL EATER'S
BOOK *of*
INSPIRATION

•

*90 Truths You Need to Know
to Overcome Your Food Addiction*

DEBBIE DANOWSKI, PhD

MARLOWE & COMPANY
NEW YORK

THE EMOTIONAL EATER'S BOOK OF INSPIRATION:
90 Truths You Need to Know to Overcome Your Food Addiction

Copyright © 2007 by Debbie Danowski, PhD
Foreword © 2007 by Phil Werdell, MA

Published by
Marlowe & Company
An Imprint of Avalon Publishing Group, Incorporated
245 West 17th Street · 11th Floor
New York, NY 10011-5300

Disclaimer:

The information in this book is intended to help readers make informed decisions about their
health and the health of their loved ones. It is not intended to be a substitute for treatment by
or the advice and care of a professional health-care provider. While the author and publisher
have endeavored to ensure that the information presented is accurate and up-to-date, they are
not responsible for adverse effects or consequences sustained by any persons using this book.

Library of Congress Cataloging-in-Publication Data
Danowski, Debbie, 1965–
    The emotional eater's book of inspiration : 90 truths you need to know
to overcome your food addiction / Debbie Danowski.
        p. cm.
    ISBN-10: 1-56924-256-9
    1. Compulsive eating—Popular works. 2. Food habits—Psychological
aspects—Popular works. 3. Weight loss—Psychological aspects—Popular
works. 4. Self-help techniques. I. Title.
RC552.C65D35 2007
616.85'26—dc22

                                                              2006026837

ISBN-13: 978-1-56924-256-8

9 8 7 6 5 4 3 2 1

Designed by Pauline Neuwirth, Neuwirth & Associates, Inc.

Printed in the United States of America

*For Charlie, who has taught me more about love
than anyone I've ever known. I love you dearly.*

•

CONTENTS

FOREWORD BY PHIL WERDELL, MA   xv
INTRODUCTION   xvii

1. *Your calendar is making you fat.*   I

2. *Simple is not the same as easy.*   4

3. *"Food lies" cause emotional eating.*   6

4. *Closing your mouth really does work.*   8

5. *What you eat should be about nutrition, not guilt.*   10

6. *A food survival pack is necessary.*   12

7. *If food calls your name, you don't have to answer.*   15

8. *Your body is more than your face.*   17

9. *You can choose your own body size.*   20

10. *Real women come in all shapes and sizes— not just 2 and 4.*   22

11. *The perfect diet doesn't exist.*   24

12. There's no such thing as a good excuse. 26

13. You need friends who understand your struggles with food. 28

14. Your own frozen dinners are better for you than any you can buy. 30

15. You are not to blame for your weight problem. 32

16. A food-free room at holiday gatherings will keep you sane. 34

17. You are not a human garbage disposal. 36

18. Cleaning your plate will not feed one single starving child. 38

19. For emotional eaters, the grocery store can be a war zone. 40

20. "Free" food is too expensive. 42

21. The space in front of the refrigerator is a "no parking" zone. 44

22. Your body is a miracle, no matter what your size. 46

23. Photographs of yourself are extremely valuable. 48

24. You can survive the "Bermuda Triangle." 50

25. Your survival depends on knowing exactly what you are eating. 53

26. Asking for help is a sign of strength not weakness. 55

27. You won't lose weight by rubbing up against a thin person. 57

28. You won't lose one ounce by talking about it. 59

29. Others are not to blame for your weight problem.   61

30. Rachael Ray doesn't eat everything she cooks and neither should you.   63

31. Cooking shows can trigger a binge.   65

32. For emotional eaters, cookbooks can be dangerous if not used correctly.   67

33. You don't need to make one more celebrity richer by buying his/her diet book.   69

34. Most models and actresses eat too little and exercise too much.   71

35. There is no law that requires you to eat chocolate on holidays.   73

36. Exercising is simply moving your body once a day.   75

37. Monday isn't the only day to begin a healthy eating plan.   77

38. There is no magical weight that will make your life perfect.   79

39. Your imperfections are a part of you.   81

40. It's what you do after a slip that matters most.   83

41. Your ideal body may not be your reality.   85

42. If your hands are busy, you won't reach for food.   87

43. You can't handle your feelings alone.   89

44. No one can lose weight for you.   91

45. Not all magazines send negative body image messages.   93

46. You're not the only one hurt by your emotional eating.   95

47. *You can accept your body with childlike wonder.* 97

48. *No one will die if you say no to dessert.* 99

49. *The food pyramid was created for a reason (and it's not to torment you).* 101

50. *Food manufacturers weren't joking when they outlined serving sizes.* 103

51. *It is best to decide what to eat when you are full.* 105

52. *Brutal honesty about your feelings won't hurt anyone.* 108

53. *Wearing big clothes only makes you look bigger.* 110

54. *Weighing yourself too often puts your emotions on the scale.* 113

55. *Food doesn't have to be on every guest list.* 115

56. *Jokes about your body size are not funny.* 117

57. *No amount of makeup can hide puffiness in your face.* 119

58. *Searching for the magic pill will prevent you from recovering.* 121

59. *Dieting is not a competitive sport.* 123

60. *Hunger pains won't kill you.* 125

61. *Having only one size of clothing in your closet keeps you honest.* 127

62. *Your too-small bathing suit is holding you captive.* 129

63. *You do deserve an occasional reward.* 131

64. *Hurting yourself even in subtle ways affects your eating.* 133

65. *The rewards matter more than the difficulties.* 135

66. *Inspiration may be corny, but it works.*   137

67. *Pretending to join the Army will save your life.*   139

68. *Standing up straight and holding your head high will make you feel confident.*   141

69. *You don't need to impersonate the Invisible Man.*   143

70. *Pleasing people by eating something is about you, not them.*   146

71. *Not acknowledging your beauty each day is an ugly thing.*   148

72. *Magic wands don't work.*   150

73. *Writing is the right thing to do.*   152

74. *Saying no is an essential part of your healing.*   154

75. *Commercials will cause cravings.*   157

76. *Baking is not a way to show love.*   159

77. *Calories don't count.*   161

78. *Food funerals help you to mourn.*   163

79. *Guilt doesn't hurt as much as resentment.*   166

80. *Enjoying what you eat is not the same as eating everything you enjoy.*   169

81. *A SWAT team will rescue you.*   171

82. *Models may look good in print, but they don't look that good in reality.*   173

83. *You can't have your cake and lose weight, too.*   176

84. *Just like Linus, you will need a blanket.*   178

85. *Using food in the décor of your home is like playing with a loaded gun.*   181

86. *Love is all you need.*   183

87. *Emotional hunger isn't physical and shouldn't be treated that way.*   185

88. *Burning something will light a fire under your recovery.*   187

89. *Growing pains are part of life.*   190

90. *You are worth it.*   192

RESOURCES   194

ACKNOWLEDGMENTS   197

FOREWORD

By the year 2010, it is estimated that 40 percent of all Americans or 68 million people will be classified as obese. Currently, that figure is 31 percent. In addition, approximately 1.7 billion people worldwide should lose weight, according to the International Obesity Task Force. More than $117 billion a year is spent on obesity-related diseases for about 129 million adults in the United States who are overweight or obese, according to a report issued by Health and Human Services Secretary Tommy Thompson.

Emotional eating is the reason for many of these problems. Most of us are unaware of the ways we use food to soothe our feelings. While food addicts need to begin by abstaining from their binge foods, feelings come up especially strong when they do. Without help, it is nearly impossible to permanently change eating patterns and overcome emotional eating.

The Emotional Eater's Book of Inspirations: 90 Truths You Need to Know to Overcome Your Food Addiction is a unique and special approach to help with this problem. Denial is the number one reason many of us fail to recover; the ninety truths in this book will not only help you recognize this critical issue, they have the potential to be life-changing.

As someone who has spent all of his professional life working in the eating disorders field, I have witnessed firsthand the challenges of recovery. This book will help you through the toughest days and will be a companion as you overcome your emotional eating.

PHIL WERDELL, MA
Program Director,
ACORN Food Dependency Recovery Services
Cofounder, Food Addiction Institute

INTRODUCTION

MY HEART WAS pounding as I reached for the phone. I knew instantly something was wrong. No one ever called me this early and anyone who would knew that I had flown in from Florida the day before. I had made it clear that I planned to sleep in.

"Hello," my voice was groggy.

"Deb, it's Dad. You gotta come down to Florida. Mom is dead." I could hear the sobs in his voice.

"Oh, my God, Daddy. What happened? I'm so sorry." I was sobbing, too.

My parents were two weeks into a month-long vacation in Daytona Beach. I had just returned from visiting them. Other than a stomachache, my mother had had no symptoms when I saw her the morning before.

With shaking hands, I hung up the phone and began to prepare to fly back to Florida. Turning on the light, I saw the watch that my mother had gotten me a few days before. She had smiled at me when she found the wide pink-banded watch. She knew it was my favorite color and that I would love it.

Cradling the watch and rocking back and forth, I began to sob uncontrollably. Up until this point, I had been too young to understand the finality of death.

This time I knew. I knew that I would never again see or talk to my mother. I knew that she would never be there to listen to me talk about my problems or to offer support. And most of all, I knew that she would never be there to hug me and offer comfort in my most painful times. Now, when I needed her most she was gone.

It's been nearly two years since I received that phone call. During the time that followed, I experienced more pain than I could ever have imagined. There were endless nights of lying awake sobbing uncontrollably, the intense feelings of loneliness, and the overwhelming struggle to continue working my food addiction recovery program at all times and without exception.

Eighteen years ago, eating was the only way I knew to comfort myself. I put on a happy face then when I was alone and ate until I was so sick that I could barely make it to the bathroom in time. I was 328 pounds. Though this was painful, it didn't even compare to the deep self-hatred and shame I felt from not being able to control my eating. I felt completely defeated and demoralized each time I tried yet another diet only to end up heavier than when I began. I was suicidal and hopeless.

And though I needed to be locked up in a treatment center to begin my recovery that is not true for everyone. As someone who is physically addicted to processed sugar and flour in the same way that an alcoholic is to alcohol, I needed to find a food plan that worked for me. I did. But this was only the first step.

Having a food plan that allowed me to be free of my addictive substances allowed my true feelings to surface. For the first time in my life I was able to identify what I was feeling. Before this, I had spent so much time and energy eating that I wasn't aware of my emotions. Once I could identify them, I needed to learn what to do with them. Since eating had been my only course of action before, I had to change many things in my life.

Today, I am happy to say that I am able to feel my feelings and not use food to deny them. Even in extreme cases such as the death of my mother, I know that no amount of food can take away the pain I am feeling. In fact, it is exactly the opposite. If I do choose to reach for food when I have strong feelings then I will experience even more pain than if I had let myself experience them.

Now, it's your turn. Picking up this book is an indication that you are probably experiencing some degree of pain due to your connection to food. Maybe you are like I was and suicidal, or perhaps you just have fleeting thoughts of wanting to improve your eating habits. Whatever the degree of your problem, it's important that you begin to take responsibility for finding a solution.

This book will help you to do that. Within these pages you will find 90 truths to help you overcome your emotional eating and food addiction. You will be offered concrete activities to help you both identify your feelings and improve your eating habits. But, most of all you will learn new ways of managing your emotions so that you no longer need to use food to make yourself feel better.

One of the important things I've learned to recognize in my own recovery is how I used "food lies" to allow myself to continue my emotional eating. Throughout this book you will learn to identify and change the food lies you have created to sustain your over- or undereating. You will be presented with workable methods of moving forward and creating a happy and sane life.

Before you begin, there are a few things you need to know. The terms food addiction and emotional eating are used throughout this book. It is important to understand the difference. "Food addiction" is a term used to describe a physical and emotional addiction to certain food substances, usually processed sugar, flour, caffeine, sometimes fats and wheat. "Emotional eating" is used to label the condition of using food to manage feelings. While all food addicts are emotional eaters, not all emotional eaters are food addicts. In other words, it is possible to emotionally eat without being physically addicted to food.

It is also important to note that not all food addicts and emotional eaters are overweight. There are many forms of both. A person can be addicted to food yet abstain from eating. It's not how much or how little a person eats, it's what the food does to the person that matters. Some emotional eaters and food addicts feel powerful by not eating. When they do eat, they feel out of control.

With all of the varieties of both food addiction and emotional eating, it is best that you try not to compare yourself to others. Rather than dismissing things that may not initially seem to fit your circumstances, take some time to make every effort to identify with the things written in this book. Put all thoughts about how you are different out of your mind. Instead, think about those things that do pertain to you. It will make all of the difference in the world in determining the progress you will make.

The next thing you need to understand is that this book does not offer a suggested food plan. You will need to find one. How you go about this is up to you. There are resources at the end of this book to help. You may use one of them or you may decide to consult a doctor or nutritionist. Whatever course you take, do not try to figure it out yourself. As an emotional eater or food addict, it is important that you have some accountability when deciding what to eat. Look at it this way, if you could have changed your eating habits by yourself then you wouldn't be where you are now.

As you read the entries and work on the suggested activities, understand that the single most important trait you bring to beginning this book is honesty. If you're like many emotional eaters and food addicts you have spent a lifetime telling yourself food lies so that you can over- or undereat. Being 100 percent honest about food and your feelings is a challenge but it is necessary.

And, finally, it will be helpful for you to purchase a special notebook or journal where you can keep all your thoughts about your recovery in one place. Though some people are resistant to do this because they are afraid that someone will find their writings, understand that with any type of recovery there are risks and challenges. If this is a particular challenge for you, then take every precaution you can to store your journal in a safe place. At the same time, understand that some people use this as an excuse not to move forward. If this is the case, keep in mind that your own words may save your life someday.

To begin, make a commitment to yourself to read one entry and complete the suggested activity each day for the next 90 days. Set aside a designated time that works for you. For some people it is first thing in the morning, while for others it is after work or before bed. The time doesn't matter nearly as much as consistency.

The program here is designed to build upon what you learn every day. Though you may be tempted to read the whole book all at once then put it down, I recommend that you stick to reading one entry each day for the next 90 days. After you've finished 90 days, you can and should dip into the book when you need a reminder to stick with your new eating habits.

If you are experiencing an extremely difficult time you may choose to read or reread some of the other entries but be sure not to skip over any of the activities when you do get to them. In other words, it's okay to read the entries out of order if you need to but make every effort to read and complete the activities in order.

Keep reading and whatever you do, don't stop. Don't talk yourself out of continuing. Turn the page and move forward into the life that you've always dreamed of. I know this is possible. I am living proof and it is my hope that someday you will be, too.

1

Your calendar is making you fat.

IT MAY SEEM unbelievable that the first and most important step in beginning a sensible eating journey has nothing to do with food. But if you think about it for a minute, it begins to make sense. How many times have you become discouraged because you weren't losing weight fast enough? And what did you do when you became frustrated? Let me guess: eat.

One of the biggest mistakes most emotional eaters make is to plan their weight loss. How many times have you tried to lose weight in anticipation of that big party in a few months? Or any other big event taking place on a designated date? What happened when you didn't reach your goal? The party came and went just as planned. If you did lose weight, then chances are you returned to your former eating behavior shortly after the event. The calendar served as both a beginning and ending point.

Your journey into healthy eating must not be dependent on calendars and timetables. It must become a daily way of life.

The truth is that no matter how much planning we do, the weight will come off in our body's time, not our calendar's. Weight loss is proportionate to the types and quantities of food we eat and the exercise we do, not to the amount of time we spend planning it.

Planning our weight loss only makes us frustrated and angry when we don't reach our goals, or cocky and celebratory when we do. Either way leads us back to overeating. The time will pass no matter what, but how we spend that time is up to us. Do we really want to be disillusioned by our lofty weight-loss goals, or would we rather be taking steps toward reaching a healthy weight?

When I weighed over 300 pounds, each time I began a new diet I would plan to lose five pounds a week. That meant that in less than half a year I would lose 100 of the 150 pounds I needed to. Inevitably, I fell short of my goal within a matter of weeks.

Since I had failed to reach my goal, I figured I may as well quit altogether. Why bother to stick to a diet if I couldn't even do something as simple as lose five pounds a week? I went back to my unhealthy eating habits and added even more weight to my already enormous body size, which eventually prolonged the amount of time I would actually need once I began to lose weight.

Had I thrown my calendar away, I would not have set myself up to fail before I even began. And that's the main reason for throwing away our calendars—to prevent us from becoming too attached to unrealistic goals that are impossible to meet.

So, go ahead! Forget planning your weight loss. Stop putting so much pressure on yourself. Your first task in this program is to throw away your calendar. Open up that garbage can immediately! Your body, and your mind, will thank you.

2

Simple is not the same as easy.

Overcoming emotional eating and food addiction is simple. Simple? Yes. It's a matter of eating nutritious foods, exercising, avoiding processed sugar and flour, and eating moderate meals. There's no magic to it. It isn't brain surgery. It's quite simple. Even a five-year-old can understand the concept.

The problem is that as simple as the idea is, the execution of it is not easy. Many of us are trying to change years of both family and societal conditioning. We have been taught that food makes everything better; that eating cupcakes is the way to celebrate a child's birthday; that baking your grandmother cookies will make her feel cared for; that eating ice cream will soothe a broken heart; and that fast food is a way to give yourself a break.

We value thin, lean bodies but we gorge ourselves with high calorie foods to soothe our emotions. We have been trained to strive for an unrealistic physical ideal while at the same time treating ourselves to foods that have no real nutritional value. Fighting these contradictory messages is no easy task. And the battle must be waged on both an emotional and physical level.

Physically, if you haven't already done so, you will need to find a food plan that works for you. To do this, you may want to consult with a nutritionist who is skilled at helping food addicts, refer to a book written to address the physical issues, or attend a workshop. See the Resources Section in the back of the book for suggestions.

Emotionally, it will be necessary to detach from food. You will need to view food as simply a means of nourishing your body rather than soothing your emotions. Though this is a challenging process it is not impossible. But make no mistake. It will take work. You cannot simply read this book and hope to magically overcome your emotional eating. You will need to actually complete the activities in each entry. You will need to put effort and time into your recovery program. And no one else can do that for you.

As you take your first steps to free yourself from emotional eating, make a decision to commit a certain amount of time each day to work on this program. Spend your time today thinking about how you can rearrange your schedule to find fifteen minutes each day to focus on your new lifestyle. Set aside this time in the same way that you would a doctor or dentist appointment. This is your time and nothing should get in the way. It may not be easy but it is necessary.

3

"Food lies" cause emotional eating.

━━━

Just one won't hurt.
I really don't eat that much.
My body size doesn't bother me.
There really aren't that many calories in that.

THESE ARE EXAMPLES of "food lies": things we tell ourselves to keep us from knowing the truth about our eating. The easiest way to continue emotionally eating is to
believe these lies. The only way we can allow ourselves to
continue doing something we know is so harmful to our
bodies is to lie to ourselves and, in some cases, to others.

Almost from the time we are born, food plays an emotional role in our lives. If a baby cries, parents assume she's
hungry and offer bottles. As we get older, we are often
rewarded for good behavior with lollipops or candy. This
cements the association between food and love from an
early age.

We are trained to use food to make us feel better yet somewhere along the line, food turns on us. It stops working. We no longer feel good after we eat, and in a misguided attempt to capture those good feelings, we continue to eat more and more. We know deep inside of us that eating isn't doing what we want it to yet we still keep hoping that we can fill the emptiness inside of us with food.

If you want to change things then you will need to recognize the food lies you've come to believe. To do this, you first have to be clear about what these lies are. The four listed above only scratch the surface. You will have your own personal food lies and they may not match any of those mentioned here.

Usually, you will notice the food lies surfacing right before you reach for food. Rather than eat, take a second to write down your thoughts. What words are you using to justify your eating?

Once you have identified your thoughts, it will be necessary to write the "healthy truths" that go along with them. For example, I combat the food lie *Just one won't hurt* with the truth that *Eating one will lead to eating the whole bag. I really don't eat that much?* The truth here is that *I am probably eating more than I think.* Now, it's your turn. Make the list and turn your food lies into food truths.

4

Closing your mouth really does work.

CAN OVERCOMING EMOTIONAL eating really be as simple as closing your mouth? Yes! Think about what it would be like if every time you wanted to eat something you closed your mouth. Then, imagine if you only opened your mouth for nutritious food at specific meal times.

Remember the difference between simple and easy? Though the suggestion above may seem too simple, it does work. And it can be easy. A big part of the denial that exists in emotional eaters involves a lack of honesty. Many times the denial is so strong that we actually aren't even aware of some of the things we are eating. Many studies have shown that underreporting food intake is common in overweight people. In other words, the people in these studies aren't aware of how many times they actually opened their mouths.

Start by making an agreement with yourself. Decide that you will only open your mouth to eat four times per day. For example, I begin my day by eating breakfast then wait four or five hours for lunch, then four or five hours for dinner, and later have a small snack before bed. If you eat breakfast at 8:00 AM then lunch would be at 12:00 or 1:00 PM, dinner at 5:00 PM and snack at 9:00 PM. (This plan may not be right for you, so you may want to consult a nutritionist or a registered dietician to develop your own program.) Besides the times mentioned, your mouth is closed for eating.

Think of it like a business. There are designated hours that the store is open and hours that it isn't. Your mouth is the same. Your mouth is not a 24-hour/7-days-a-week convenience. Instead, your hours are clear and you must stick to them. At any other time your mouth is closed.

Today, make your own schedule of the hours your mouth will be open. If you feel like eating during other times, picture a huge sign with orange letters saying closed. You wouldn't dream of going into a business that was closed. It's the same for your mouth.

5

*What you eat should be about nutrition,
not guilt.*

It was POPCORN and potato chips for me. I craved the
crunchy saltiness of potato chips but told myself that they
were too high in calories so I chose "low" calorie popcorn
to alleviate the guilt I would feel if I actually ate what I really
wanted. The problem was that I ate twice as much popcorn
to make up for not having the potato chips. The guilt and
anger I felt about overeating actually worked against me,
beginning a vicious cycle that lasted for years.

Had I learned how to make food choices based on my
body's nutritional needs, I would have saved myself many
hours of anguish as well as years of weight gain. And I
wouldn't have chosen either popcorn or potato chips.
When we feed our body what it *needs*, we remove guilt
from the eating experience.

One of the ways many of us trick ourselves into overeating is by substituting what seems to be less "dangerous"
food. Rather than eating a little of what we really crave, we
eat a lot more of the less desirable food. All the while we tell

ourselves how guilty we feel for eating at all when we are angry that we aren't eating the food we really want.

The healthy truth here is that eating is intended to be a means of nourishing our bodies. It is not a way to make ourselves feel better or a method to deal with guilt. If we eat what we know is healthy and good for our bodies, we banish the shame that comes with overeating or choosing foods that we know will cause us to gain weight.

Even though we may believe otherwise, the healthy truth is that eating what is good for our bodies is actually easier than choosing foods that we know will harm us. Today, make a choice to eat nutritious foods. Think about all of the guilt and anger you'll avoid by making a decision to change.

6

A food survival pack is necessary.

▄ ▄

I had to eat what was there.
But there wasn't anything healthy . . .
This is what they're serving.

THESE ARE SOME common food lies we tell ourselves
when we are away from home. The healthy truth here is
that the only truly safe foods are the ones that you prepare
yourself. You will need to carry a food survival pack. With
your new way of thinking, you must eliminate all of the
food lies you tell yourself. As you move forward, you will
need to realize that there is no excuse good enough to
make you eat unhealthy foods.

Over time, we have become so good at blaming others
or making them responsible for our food choices that we
fail to admit our own responsibility. Instead of using
excuses about the types of foods that are absent, we need
to get honest about our true motives. Many of us attend

special gatherings as an excuse to overeat. We believe that if we are out of our own kitchens then we have no responsibility for the food we consume.

Similarly, we tell ourselves that if we are at a restaurant we must eat what everyone else chooses and that we must make the most of our evening out. The problem is that this kind of thinking gives you a license to eat whatever you want without considering the consequences.

Every ounce of food you eat contributes to either the health or the destruction of your body. As much as you may wish to eat whatever you want when you're out without gaining weight, this is not going to happen. When you eat food that's been prepared at a restaurant or for a special occasion, chances are it's higher in calories and fat. Instead of thinking about food that you eat out as not counting in your daily consumption, consider it twice as dangerous.

Carrying a food survival pack will take away any excuses you may have to eat foods high in calories and fat. Instead of saying, "They didn't have anything healthy," you can eat the food you brought. A food survival pack also means bringing your own lunch or dinner to work or school so that you have healthy food to eat.

What you put into your food survival pack should be based on your individual healthy eating plan. But, you need to be careful not to carry an overabundance of food with you since this, too, can be a setup to overeat. Some ideas include: sugar-free, low-fat salad dressing, fresh vegetables, canned vegetables, salad, and tuna. It may take some extra work but it is worth the effort. Today, put together your own food survival pack. You can stop telling yourself food lies and start taking responsibility.

7

If food calls your name,
you don't have to answer.

"I'M HERE!" THE words were loud. "Come and get me. I'll taste so good." It was the half gallon of chocolate chip ice cream in the freezer. "Think about how creamy I am." The words chanted in my head over and over again until I could no longer resist. Running to the refrigerator, I grabbed the ice cream then a spoon and began to shove spoonfuls into my mouth. I didn't stop until it was all gone. My stomach ached and I was nauseous. Even worse, I was humiliated. I hated myself for being so weak.

Despite what we may think, food cannot speak to us. It does not breathe. It is not living and we cannot hurt its feelings if we don't eat it. These are just excuses that we use to overeat.

By giving human characteristics to food we create a relationship with an object. Once we create this relationship we become emotionally attached to it. This allows us to manufacture situations that make it nearly impossible for us to resist overeating. In a sense, we are using food to replace the human relationships that involve the person who once served them to us.

Most times when we feel as if food is calling out to us it is because we are experiencing strong emotions that we don't want to deal with. We don't want to experience our feelings so we turn to food to help us feel better. We make ourselves believe that food is calling out to us so that we can rationalize eating things that we know are unhealthy.

The best course of action when you feel as if food is calling your name is to run, walk, or move your body in some way. Rather than make a beeline for the refrigerator, walk out the door and to the park. Take a few minutes to sit outside on the porch or grab your golf clubs and go. If the weather doesn't allow this then take a walk inside the house or go to the mall. Whatever it is that works for you, do it.

Today, don't give your mind one second more to actually believe that food is calling your name. Remind yourself that food doesn't speak and that even if it did, you don't have to listen. You can choose to walk away instead.

8

Your body is more than your face.

■ ■ ■

"YOU'VE GOT SUCH a pretty face . . ." The words are spoken then there's a pause. The rest of the sentence, ". . . it's too bad about the rest of your body," often remains unsaid even though we all know it's there. Whether or not you have been on the receiving end of this sentiment, there is a good chance that you are saying the same thing to yourself.

How many times have you looked in the mirror only to see your face rather than your entire body? Do you even own a full-length mirror or are you deceiving yourself by seeing only what's above your neck?

Some of us may be feeling a bit overwhelmed by the thought of looking in a full-length mirror. We may be thinking that seeing what we truly look like will cause more harm than good, that we will only end up hating ourselves even more.

It's important to understand that a look in the mirror should give us a realistic picture of ourselves, not a means to criticize ourselves. Even though this may seem impossible there are a few things you can do to make viewing your reflection a more positive experience.

To begin, understand that negative thoughts will come up. Many of us have been trained since early childhood to view our bodies critically. Negative thoughts are normal. But, you don't have to listen to them. Instead, you can simply let the words float in to your head then right out. You don't have to fight them and you don't have to believe them. You can simply accept them as part of your makeup, all the while knowing that these ideas aren't true.

When you look in the mirror, you may feel sad at first. This is only natural considering that you have probably ignored and/or vilified your body for years. At this point, you may feel so vulnerable for exposing yourself in this way that feeling sad is to be expected. Let the feeling wash over you all the while realizing that you will not die from sadness.

After the sadness passes, take a few minutes to look at every part of your body. Notice your neck, your shoulders, your arms, your chest, your waist, your hips, your legs, even your feet. Though there may be areas that you are not satisfied with, put those thoughts aside for the moment. Instead, look at each area and find something that you like about it. Come up with a few nice thoughts about each area of your body.

For instance, is your neck long, your arms strong, your shoulders broad, or your hips sturdy? Do you have pretty hands or glamorous feet? Are your legs physically power-ful or is your body nicely proportionate? Let the thoughts flow into your mind. Savor the newness of saying nice things about your body. Though it may be uncomfortable, realize the more you do it the healthier your body image will become.

Don't give up no matter how it feels. Simply trust that when you look in the mirror below your neck, you will ultimately develop a realistic image of your body that will allow you to become honest about your life and your eating.

9

You can choose your own body size.

REMEMBER THOSE INSURANCE height and weight charts? How many times have you used them to make yourself feel badly about your body size? Did you tell yourself that you weren't thin enough, which then led you to seek solace in high calorie foods?

Even though these charts were developed as a means to determine healthy body weights, they can actually cause distress for those of us who struggle with body image issues. Many times the numbers seem so low that we feel it is impossible for us to reach them so we simply give up and continue to overeat.

What we need to do instead is stop looking at the numbers and concentrate on eating healthy, well-balanced meals. If we are vigilant about doing this, the weight will take care of itself.

After nearly twenty years of maintaining a 160-pound weight loss, the numbers on my scale are still on the high side of these charts. I never reached what would be considered my "goal" weight. Instead, my body stabilized at a reasonable weight, though not the number the insurance charts had touted as my ideal weight. Despite the fact that I have had plastic surgery to remove hanging skin from my stomach and my upper arms, I still have hanging skin on my legs, butt, and hips. There aren't any weight charts to account for this.

And even though I can move around in ways that I only once dreamed about when I weighed 328 pounds, whenever I look at the charts that describe my ideal weight I feel inadequate. I sometimes even beat up on myself. The difference today is that I know I get to choose my body size. Rather than falling prey to unrealistic or inappropriate weight charts, I can choose to appreciate the uniqueness of my body.

Even though I did not reach my "ideal" weight, I did consult with several people to make sure that I was being realistic about the numbers on the scale. By getting honest with others, I allowed myself the dignity of choosing a weight that worked for me without the danger of denying an unhealthy situation. I didn't allow choosing my own body size as a means to deny my emotional eating problem either. Now it's your turn. Today, choose a weight that works for you and be proud that you have the choice. No one has the right to tell you what you should weigh. That's *your* job.

10

Real women come in all shapes and sizes—not just 2 and 4.

Y OU'VE SEEN THEM on television and on glossy pages. They sneak into your home and taunt you with their "perfect" bodies. Program after program, magazine cover after magazine cover, these models proudly show off every slender curve of their bodies, the whole time smiling beautifully. How can you possibly compete?

The answer is simple—you can't. And, even more, you shouldn't even try. Instead, your energy would be better spent understanding the way these images are created. To begin with, 99 percent of the models you see on magazine covers have been digitally altered and, in some cases, given entirely new bodies.

In a recent article in *Glamour* magazine, a television actress outlined the digital alteration process that includes shaving a few inches off of her already slender hips, erasing blemishes, under eye circles, and cellulite.

Keep in mind that this is someone who makes her living looking extraordinarily beautiful. Even she needs help to appear the way you see her in a magazine. What does this mean for the rest of us?

It's impossible to look like the women you see on television and in magazines and you shouldn't try. Read that again: It's impossible to look like the women you see on television and in magazines and you shouldn't try.

In reality, holding these images up as ideal for our own bodies is a form of denial. The food lie goes like this: *Since I can't look like* _____ *(fill in the blank), then I will give up and eat whatever I want.* These perfect bodies become our excuses to overeat.

Rather than use them to beat yourself up, you can instead make a decision to view these images as you would a painting—very beautiful, requiring tremendous amounts of work, and not something 99 percent of us can achieve. Your goal here is to be in the best shape that *your* body can be, not someone else's.

Today, give up the idea of living up to the media's unrealistic standards and work toward having a healthy body. You'll be amazed at how freeing it will be to stop beating yourself up for something that not only is out of reach, but unhealthy for you as well.

11

The perfect diet doesn't exist.

WHAT DO YOU really want? A diet that will let you eat everything you crave and lose weight?

Let's get honest—this doesn't exist. If you want to lose weight you will need to eat nutritious foods and exercise. There is no magic involved.

Looking for the perfect diet is a way to pretend you are taking action when you really aren't. You can busy yourself with this task rather than having to change your eating habits. The search allows you to continue over- or undereating.

Trying to find the perfect diet is a way to prolong taking action. In theory, it seems as if you are actually moving forward yet you are stuck in seeking what you believe will be the answer to all of your problems. The healthy truth here is that the answers you are seeking have to come from within you.

Rather than looking for something outside of yourself (a diet), you need to develop the inner strength to take steps that will allow you to overcome your emotional eating. The food plan isn't nearly as important as your resolve to follow it.

This is where the time comes to make choices that will support ending your emotional eating. For instance, the next time you want to reach for ice cream when you are upset, call a friend instead. If you're tempted by chocolate cake, take a walk or read a book. Do whatever you have to so that you don't reach for food. That's the way you will change your eating habits—by taking action and making yourself vulnerable to new ways of doing things. The perfect diet has little to do with this.

If you are a food addict, however, you will need to find a plan that does not include your addictive substances. But even a plan that addresses these issues isn't "the perfect diet." While "the perfect diet" doesn't exist, sticking to a sensible plan and staying true to your goals will help you overcome your emotional eating and lead a life you never thought was possible.

12

There's no such thing as a good excuse.

IF YOU TRULY want to eat healthier then you have no business being around foods that don't fit into that lifestyle. It's just that simple. There's no need to torture yourself or romanticize foods that you don't eat. We would never think about putting our hand on a hot burner yet we continually do the very same thing where food is concerned.

We tell ourselves things such as: *I can handle it* or *It's rude if I don't have any.* Let's be clear: These are simply the food lies we tell ourselves to be around food. For many of us food is our best friend, our lover, and even our confidant. Because of this we love being around it. We get a certain emotional high from spending time with the love of our lives in the same way that we do when we are near people we love.

Unlike the people we love, however, being around food is dangerous for us. We don't need to pretend to be strong. We don't need to expose ourselves to things that will harm us. We especially don't need to sit there and watch others eat high calorie desserts. And, we certainly don't need to make others feel wrong or bad for choosing to eat things that we don't.

Here's one solution to all of this: Leave the table when dessert is served. If you are at a restaurant, simply go to the bathroom. If you're at someone's house, you can also use the bathroom, but you can also take a walk around the block, help with the dishes, or go into another room. It doesn't matter what you decide to do as long as you leave the area where the dessert is.

Don't fool yourself into believing that you will be strong this time. Even if you do manage to make it through this meal without eating dessert, chances are that you will try to "reward" yourself with another dessert shortly after. Once the idea of dessert is put into your mind, it's a good bet that you will begin to romanticize the food, which will eventually lead to eating it.

Rather than trying to be strong enough to handle being around the dessert, realize that real strength lies in knowing your limits. Today, make a plan to go to the bathroom when dessert is served. You'll be amazed at how well this will work for you.

13

*You need friends who understand
your struggles with food.*

As I sit here writing this I want to eat something that I know isn't good for me. It's been an extremely emotional week. My father was diagnosed with cancer and my relationship of a year and a half ended abruptly and painfully.

Of course, the first place I want to run is right to the refrigerator. The funny thing about all of this is that for one of the first times in my life I don't feel like eating. I am sick with emotion and the core of this sickness is in my stomach. I just want something to make myself feel better.

The problem is that I know nothing can. No one can swoop in and remove all of my pain. But I do know something that has helped—having friends who understand and support me in my struggles with both food and life.

When I weighed over 300 pounds, I didn't have many friends. All I wanted to do was eat and I pushed everyone away to do that. Today, nearly twenty years later, my life is completely different. Though I resisted letting people into my life and sometimes still do, I have come to realize that I can't get through my life alone.

For me, this means being a member of many different kinds of support groups. I attend one group that helps me with my food issues, another that helps me with relationship issues, one for my spirituality, and still another for my writing. And though this may seem like a lot, and maybe it is, my life is completely different than it was seventeen years ago.

After I was divorced three years ago, I realized that I had pushed most of the people in my life away in a misguided attempt to save my marriage. I had to go out and make it a point to meet people by attending events in my community, signing up for lectures, and reaching out to others. It wasn't easy, and having friends doesn't solve all of my problems, but it does make life a lot more manageable.

Today, even though my pain is overwhelming, there are people in my life who remind me that over- or undereating will not make anything better, that my pain has a beginning and an ending, and that I will survive this no matter how much I think I won't.

Why don't you try it? Today, make it a point to say hello to at least two people you have never greeted before. Who knows? It could be the start of a beautiful friendship.

14

Your own frozen dinners are better for you than any you can buy.

I don't have time to cook nutritious food.
I need quick meals.

How MANY TIMES have you told yourself these things as you reached for high calorie fast food? One of the ways that we fool ourselves into eating unhealthy foods is by using the food lie that we are too busy to prepare something nutritious. It is much easier to drive through a fast food restaurant or pull out a frozen dinner, we tell ourselves.

The healthy truth is that it takes just as much time and effort to go to the restaurant or store to buy and prepare the high calorie foods as it does to cook healthy food. We only tell ourselves how difficult making nutritious food is as a way to justify eating fat-filled items. In other words, lack of time is simply an excuse.

One of the ways to make it easier for yourself is to prepare healthy meals in advance. By making your own frozen dinners, you will have appropriate, tasty food readily available. While you may be tempted to completely dismiss this idea, take a moment to think about the benefits.

In as little as an hour you can have all the meals you need for an entire week. This means that not only would you be able to simply pull a nutritious, tasty prepared meal out the freezer and heat it up but you wouldn't have to wait in line at a fast food restaurant or even deal with making an extra stop. Everything you need would already be at your fingertips.

If you're not known for your cooking skills then it may be a good idea to start with simple meals. You may also want to speak to a nutritionist to help with ideas for healthy meals. And realize that with a little practice preparing food in advance will become second nature. Today, make a plan to prepare your own frozen dinners. You are worth the initial investment of time and energy that it will take to become familiar with the process of making frozen dinners. And best of all, this will banish the food lie of not having time to prepare healthy foods.

15

You are not to blame for your weight problem.

I'm too weak.
I have no willpower.
I'm disgusting.

DOES ANY OF THIS sound familiar? Have you said these things to yourself at least once? Many times? Well, today is the day to make a different choice to actually look at why you treat yourself like this.

To begin, you need to understand how you use these thoughts to overeat. If you keep telling yourself how weak and disgusting you are then you get to feel badly. And, if you feel depressed or sad then how can you make yourself feel better? By eating, of course.

Yes, some of your choices have contributed to your current state. Beating yourself up allows you to remain stuck in a victim mode and thus continue your unhealthy lifestyle. By taking responsibility for your life you claim the power to change things.

How do you take responsibility? The first step is to become aware of your actions. How much are you over- or undereating? When do you struggle most? What seems to trigger your emotional eating? Are there social situations that seem to be more difficult eating challenges or do challenges come when you are alone? Begin to become aware of when you are most tempted to use food to soothe yourself.

After you are clear on this, try to think of ways to improve the situation. For example, if you tend to feel especially emotional at night when you are alone then either make plans with friends, pick up the phone, write, or take a walk instead of putting yourself in that position.

Today is the day you can make the decision to refuse to blame yourself for your weight problem. Instead, take responsibility and watch your life change.

16

*A food-free room at holiday gatherings
will keep you sane.*

So MANY OF us let other people make decisions for us when holiday time comes around. Rather than taking care of ourselves, we use the excuse that we have no control over what other people do. And while this may be true, the real question is how many times have we actually asked for what we needed?

If you are like most people, the answer is probably not many. Unfortunately, many of us expect other people to anticipate our needs or, even more challenging, to read our minds. Instead of making a request, we sit back and hope that others will simply do what we want them to.

Not only is this unfair and unrealistic but it is a form of self-delusion as well. By failing to ask for what you want, you place responsibility for yourself in someone else's hands. And the reality is that if you do this, you have a better chance of *not* getting the healthy food you need.

In other words, not getting nutritious food becomes someone else's fault *and* provides you with an excuse to eat items you know are harmful. For someone who is looking for an excuse to overeat, it's the best of both worlds: You don't have to take responsibility and you have someone else to blame.

If, however, your goal is to end your emotional eating then you will need to change the way you manage holiday situations. It is time for you to take responsibility for your needs. This does not mean you should demand anything but simply ask, all the while realizing that the person you are asking has the right to deny your request. In this case, you will need to come up with an alternative plan: Perhaps you can leave before the meal is served or arrive after everyone has eaten. Or, you can find a room where there isn't any food. Some people feel compelled to put snack dishes by every seat so this may be challenging for some of us. If you find the dish of chips by your chair, move the snack to another table or another room.

Whatever it is you have to do, do it. You may need to be creative but it will be worth it. And, if you do choose to overeat, realize it is your choice. No one else has done that to you. Today, make it a point to begin practicing by asking for what you need. Know that this is a way of taking responsibility for yourself. After all, mind reading is a lost art.

17

You are not a human garbage disposal.

▪▪▪

"I CAN'T LET it go to waste." How many times have you used this as an excuse to eat something that wasn't healthy for you? Many of us treat our bodies as human garbage disposals—throwing into them anything that's left over. Though this may seem financially efficient, it is physically and emotionally destructive. If we convince ourselves that all the food in our house must be eaten rather than thrown away, we give ourselves permission to eat more than our bodies need.

This type of thinking enables you to look outside of yourself to determine how much you should eat. Instead, you need to make eating decisions based on biological needs rather than the amount of food left.

For most of us, the feeling of physical hunger is an unfamiliar experience. Since we regularly eat more than our bodies need, we don't actually know what *hunger* feels like. Eating food based on emotions has caused distance from our basic physiological needs.

Take a second to think about what hunger feels like. What happens in your body? Can you describe the experience? Do you feel a rumbling in your stomach? Are you light-headed? Whatever it is, write it down then hang the list on your refrigerator. Today, read the list to make sure you are truly hungry before eating.

Truly listening to your body and refusing to treat yourself as a human garbage disposal are important steps in separating your physiological needs from your emotional wants. And though it may be frightening at first to think about only eating when you are hungry, if you are consistent, you will notice progress. Instead of being a human garbage disposal you will become a healthy and strong human being.

18

*Cleaning your plate will not feed one
single starving child.*

IN THE SAME way that being a human garbage disposal
causes you to look outside of yourself to determine how
much you eat, cleaning your plate because there are starving children does the same thing. Once again, rather
than connecting with your internal biological needs, you
are using external situations to dictate your food intake.

Leaving food on your plate does not mean you are an
ingrate or wasteful. Whether you throw the food away, save
it for another meal, or eat it yourself, you are the only person affected. Should you have the urge to help fight world
hunger, it would be best to send donations to organiza-
tions set up to help feed malnourished people.

Starving children need donations of money and food
to help them. Cleaning your plate has nothing to do with
this. The fact that you have put the two incidents together
proves exactly how powerful your denial is. In other words,
you are looking for an excuse to overeat and you've chosen starving children to help you.

Today, make a commitment to reserve 10 percent of what you would normally spend at the grocery store each month to donate to a charity that helps others. If you do this, you will no longer need to make up excuses to overeat in the name of those who have less. Instead, you will know that you are making a difference through your donations, not through your stomach.

19

*For emotional eaters, the grocery store
can be a war zone.*

How many times have you walked into the grocery
store with the intention of purchasing only one or two
items and ended up with a cart full? How often were the
items you chose high in calories and fat?

One of the most common ways that we trick ourselves into
bringing unhealthy foods into our homes is by going into
a grocery store under false pretenses. Oftentimes we
convince ourselves that we must stop and buy the item we
need immediately. Yet, chances are that rather than truly
needing that particular thing we are subconsciously planning
to buy something soothing to us.

Our minds can be quite stealthy about our true inten-
tions. Whenever I feel overwhelmingly compelled to do
something, chances are that I'm reacting out of an uncon-
scious desire that I am unaware of. The best thing I can do
for myself in a situation like this is to take a deep breath
and wait a few minutes before acting.

When it becomes vitally important that you stop at the grocery store for that one item that you believe you can't live without, take a second to really think about it. Are you feeling overly emotional? Has something happened in your life that has upset you or even made you happy?

Instead of running to the grocery store, take a few minutes to connect with your inner emotions to determine if it's food you really are craving. Would it be smarter to pick up the phone and call a friend or write down how you are feeling? Then, if you still feel as if you need to go to the grocery store at least you will have a better idea of why you are compelled to do so.

When you do enter the grocery store understand that you are entering a dangerous place and take necessary precautions. First, have a list with you and stick to it. Second, ignore all items on sale. Don't go down every aisle; stick to those areas that contain only the foods on your list. And lastly, get in and out as quickly as possible. Today, know that you don't have to enter a war zone without a battle plan.

20

"Free" food is too expensive.

FREE FOOD!!!! DOES your heart race just from reading these words? What are your first thoughts? Get as
much as you can? Throw all healthy eating rules out the
window? Calories don't count?

By now your heart is racing and you're feeling a surge
of excitement, right? Even after all of my years of healthy
eating, nothing gets my blood pumping like the idea of
free food. During my most unhealthy eating periods, I
viewed free food as having no calories. Since I didn't pay
for it then why should it count?

Since then, I've realized two things about free food.
First, most times the free food is expensive in calories and
fat. It makes sense that manufacturers offering samples or
people putting on special events want to entice you with
delicious food. To make the food taste extraordinary, gobs
of butter, oil, and/or sugar are pumped into the items.

The second thing I've learned about free food is that
there is a high price to pay for eating it. As a food addict,

if I take even one bite of sugar- or flour-filled foods I will experience uncontrollable physical cravings for more of the same. Despite my best efforts, I will end up back to where I began at 328 pounds, or even worse.

For those who are not physically addicted, the "price" is still steep. Research has shown that eating foods high in calories and fat triggers a desire for more of them. For emotional eaters, the feelings of being nurtured from free food are still difficult to resist.

There are other costs. Whenever you eat something you know is unhealthy you feel ashamed, guilty, and even disgusted. You beat yourself up and start to feel hopeless. Bite by bite you erode your self-esteem and cause even greater physical and emotional pain.

Now, knowing all of this, it's time to admit that there is no such thing as free food. So the next time your heart races at the thought simply consider the high price you will pay.

21

*The space in front of the refrigerator is a
"no parking" zone.*

Dᴵᴰ ʏᴏᴜ ᴋɴᴏᴡ that there is now a refrigerator with a
television on the front of it? Today's modern technology
allows us to have every imaginable convenience possible.
Yet, let's take a second to think about this particular one.
A television set on the refrigerator encourages us to hang
out not only in the kitchen but directly in front of an
appliance that stores our most loved food.

Think about it this way. Watching television is an activity that detaches you from your emotions. Eating does the
same thing. During both, you feel numb. Now add to this
the fact that the refrigerator holds the thing we treasure the
most: food. You experience feelings of joy, happiness, even
relaxation being in a room designed specifically for eating. You associate positive feelings with food. To enhance
these good feelings you will naturally reach for something
to eat since you are already in a room that encourages this.
Now, you have further cemented the connection between
food and feelings.

The only way to break through your denial whether or not your refrigerator contains a television is to stay away from both the appliance and the kitchen. Try to think about the kitchen and more specifically the area in front of the refrigerator as a "no parking" zone that you will pay a penalty for using.

The price of the ticket you will receive is a life of misery due to unhealthy eating habits. And the fee you will be charged is your self-respect and dignity. So, before you park yourself in front of the fridge, think about the penalty involved and get out of the kitchen!

22

Your body is a miracle,
no matter what your size.

My thighs are too big.
There's too much cellulite on my legs.
My stomach sticks out too much.

H OW MANY TIMES have you said these things or others like them? Many of us spend hours finding fault with our physical appearance all the while failing to recognize the true biological miracle we are.

Think about it for a second. Without any thought or effort on your part, blood is pumped through your body, your brain coordinates with your arms and legs to move around freely, and your eyes see the beauty that surrounds you.

With all of its biological functions, your body is a true marvel unmatched by any human-made creation. We worship technology yet we fail to recognize our own superior functioning.

When is the last time you thought about how grateful you are to be able to walk? To put your arms around those you love? To reason and think? To feel? All of these things make up the miracle of your body yet we are not encouraged to appreciate or even notice them.

Today, make a decision to change that. Write down ten things that you are grateful for about your body. These can be things as simple as the ability to breathe or as personal as your hazel eyes. Whatever it is, put it on paper and don't stop until you have at least ten.

Post your list in a place where you can see it daily. Then make an effort to read it at least once a day for the next sixty-eight days. When doing this, do not criticize your body in any way. That means it's time to stop thinking about the thighs that you feel are too heavy and the cellulite you don't like. Instead, concentrate on your biology and watch your attitude change.

23

*Photographs of yourself
are extremely valuable.*

I CAN HEAR the groans already! Don't skip this entry.
Continue reading. Many of us put a lot of energy into
avoiding having photographs taken. Whenever we see the
camera, we automatically run the other way.

Have you ever thought about why? I'm sure you've
come up with the idea that you prefer not to see yourself
in print but have you taken it a step further? If you don't
let anyone take your picture then you can continue staying in denial about what you look like so you can keep on
eating. It's similar to the old idea that if you don't see it
then it doesn't exist.

The only problem here is that the trouble *does* exist. You
wouldn't be reading this book if you didn't have some issue
with food or your body. Therefore, by choosing to show
up here you have already admitted that you are not happy
or satisfied with the way things are.

If this is the case, why not be completely honest? Take
a chance and see what you really look like. Don't rely on

other people's opinions or outdated images you have of yourself. Instead, take a deep breath, have a photo taken, and make a commitment to look at this picture of yourself at least four times a year.

And when you do look at it, be gentle with yourself. Even if you don't like what you see, realize that the fact you are looking at the photo is tremendous growth on your part. It is a beginning and you can work from there to make choices that support the changes you want in your life.

It may not be easy. And it certainly isn't fun but looking at a picture of yourself at least four times a year is necessary. Now, you know where you stand—and you can move forward from here.

24

You can survive the "Bermuda Triangle."

IT BEGINS ON Halloween then moves into Thanksgiving and finally Christmas, Hanukkah, or Kwanzaa, depending on your beliefs. The last three months of the year present emotional eaters with an incredible challenge. This is the Bermuda Triangle of holidays that occurs at the end of each year. Most emotional eaters don't survive.

Celebrating one holiday can be overwhelming. Three in less than sixty days can be deadly. First, there's the stress of preparation; then intense feelings of being around relatives or friends who we don't see daily. Next, we have the messages about cooking special desserts and meals, most of which are high in calories and fat. Add to this the fact that these special foods, associated with each holiday, are only available during this time period.

It's not hard to see how perfectly these conditions contribute to the already powerful denial mechanism present in those with eating issues. However, instead of becoming a victim of the Bermuda Triangle you can prepare so that you will survive, even thrive.

The first step is to admit that there will be a lot of food around. You may have difficulty. If you tell yourself that you will be fine you actually contribute to your denial. If you can convince yourself that you won't eat then you won't put effort into preparing *not* to overeat. This means you will most likely gorge yourself.

In reality, you are setting yourself up to overeat by failing to admit how difficult the holidays can be. It's a game that emotional overeaters and food addicts play: *I'll tell myself that everything will be okay and try really hard not to think about it.* You need to be honest with yourself to be successful.

The next step is to begin planning early. Starting on October 1, think about each holiday. If you hand out treats on Halloween, consider a healthy alternative to high calorie candy. Fruit, coins, gift certificates, stickers, pens, bookmarks—any of these will work.

Next, begin to plan for Thanksgiving. Perhaps this is the year that you take your family out to eat rather than cooking all of that food at your house. Before going to a restaurant, however, be sure to confirm that you can get nutritious foods.

If eating out isn't an option then plan your meal around foods you need. Remember, there is no law that says you must serve dessert. Also, be sure to have an escape plan. If you have to choose between leaving or overeating, understand that it is better to leave then suffer the consequences of gorging yourself. The Bermuda Triangle can be scary and difficult, but by paying attention and planning ahead, you can successfully navigate the treacherous waters.

25

*Your survival depends on knowing exactly
what you are eating.*

WRITE DOWN EVERY ounce of food you intend to eat
each day. What a drag! I can hear you grumbling now.
Writing down everything that you eat—and remember
spoonfuls and tastes count!—may not be fun, but it is
necessary. You already know that denial is the biggest
block to overcoming emotional overeating. You should
also recognize that we have built-in forgetters. No sooner
have we eaten something than it is instantly forgotten.

Our minds are trained to protect us from painful
information. Knowing how much we actually eat is ago-
nizing. We secretly believe that if we don't know how bad
it is then we can keep on eating. However, if we make note
of everything we consume then we will be forced to take
action.

You may be tempted to tell yourself that it's too hard to
keep track of everything you put in your mouth, or that your
day is just too busy. If you have a small notebook and pen
handy, either in your kitchen or in your purse/briefcase, the

actual effort involved in making a list of your daily food intake is minimal. As for time, we're probably talking about ten minutes a day.

If you find yourself resisting this idea, then take a step back and consider that what's really involved here is your unwillingness to get honest with yourself. With honesty comes responsibility. You have convinced yourself that it is easier to be too busy to write down what you eat than actually doing it.

That needs to stop now. Start right this second—that means if you are eating something while you are reading this, you need to write it down. Get a piece of paper. Put the date on it and make three columns. Write the time down in one column, the item(s) you are eating in the middle column and the way you feel in the third. Keep this list or your food notebook in your kitchen or wherever you are most likely to eat. Be sure to bring it with you if you are eating out or going to work.

There is no excuse good enough for not doing this. If you don't, you will never be able to overcome your denial. Pick up the pen now and begin. No excuses, and no denial.

26

*Asking for help is a sign of strength
not weakness.*

I can do this myself.
I don't need any help.
There's no way I'm asking anyone for anything.

I CAN HEAR you. Stop right now. I'll tell you immediately, you are wrong. There is no way to overcome your emotional eating or food addiction without some type of support. Why do you think diets fail? One of the biggest reasons is that people don't recognize how strong the need for help is.

It may be difficult, especially for those who were raised in confrontational or abusive families. But, with some guidelines anyone can learn to ask for help.

To begin, it's important to recognize that asking for help is not the same as expecting someone else to fix you. Asking for someone to sit with you for an hour when you feel sad or to talk to you on the phone for ten minutes when you want to share happy news is much different from expecting someone to make all of your pain go away. Receiving help is not about fixing or removing your pain. It is about managing your life in a way that does not readily encourage you to reach for food when feeling emotional.

Next, it's vital to understand that when you ask for help, the person whom you are making the request of has the right to refuse. And though this may hurt, you must not give up. Despite what you may think, when someone refuses to help you it is usually not personal or meant to harm you. In most cases it is about the other person. She may not have the emotional energy or time to offer assistance.

To make it easier, have a list of people who you can call when you need help. And, though friends and family members may be included, it's a good idea to have at least one, if not two, people on the list who share your problem. Perhaps you can attend a local support group, seek counseling, or even join a gym to meet others who can help you. Where you go for the help will depend on what you need at a particular time.

Finally, reframe the way you think about asking for help. Ask for help when you need it. Vulnerability is not weakness, it is a sign of strength and courage. The payoff will be the sanity and health that comes with ending your emotional eating.

27

*You won't lose weight by rubbing up
against a thin person.*

HOW DID SHE *do it? What is he eating? Can I have a copy of the
diet?* How many times have you practically assaulted someone who has lost weight to find out the "magic" answer?

Somewhere in the back of your mind is the idea that if
you just try hard enough to find out the weight loss secret
then you will be thin without any effort. Even though this
seems ridiculous and you may not want to admit it, it's true.

You don't want to do the work it takes to lose weight so
you invent other ways to lose weight without effort. Think
about how much time you've spent talking to people who
have lost weight trying to find out how they did it. And
when you were done, were you thin? Did you begin a diet
that worked for you in the long term?

Chances are that even if you did find a diet you could
stick to for a little while, it didn't last. The truth is that you
want to lose weight by simply being around a thin person,
as if their "thin magic" will rub off on you. If you're honest, you'll admit that this is about as much effort as you

want to put into losing weight. Like most of us, you want to be thin but you don't want to put any work into it.

Unfortunately, no matter how much you may want it, it doesn't work that way. Your denial convinces you to put your effort into searching for some magic formula, the perfect answer, the "code" that others have broken, rather than eating healthfully and exercising.

Today, rather than wasting time seeking out a thin person in order to figure out her secrets, use the time to take a walk or prepare a healthy meal. Take action instead of courting distraction.

28

You won't lose one ounce by talking about it.

LOSING WEIGHT TAKES effort, and that doesn't mean *talking* about it. It means *doing* something about it. In other words, shut your mouth and start taking action!

Some people mistakenly think that if they obsess or worry about something enough then the problem will magically take care of itself. Many people try to convince themselves that if they talk about starting a diet, they'll eventually lose weight.

Perhaps somewhere in the back of your mind you believe that if you talk about it enough, you will never actually have to take action. In an odd way, all of this discussion allows you to continue eating foods that are unhealthy while making others believe that you are addressing your problem. It's a form of denial that keeps you from moving forward.

The reality is that no matter how much talking you do, it will not help you to lose even one ounce. Weight loss is the result of healthy eating and regular exercise. There's nothing more to it than that, and it's time to admit it. As difficult as it may be, losing weight takes effort and hard work.

After admitting that hard work is involved, you may decide that you are not up to the task. That is your right. There is no law that says you must reduce your body size. You get to choose how you want to live; with choices, however, also come consequences.

You must be prepared to accept the repercussions when you make the choice not to reduce your body size. Some of the fallout of this choice includes high blood pressure, heart disease, difficulty moving, decreased energy, physical and emotional pain, and more.

No matter what you decide, the important thing is that you are 100 percent honest with yourself. Weight loss is hard work but it's not impossible. Try not to make it harder by being all talk and no action. So make a decision, stop talking, and start doing!

29

Others are not to blame for your weight problem.

If he didn't bring cookies into the house, I wouldn't eat them.
How can I resist her apple pie?
If she wasn't such a good cook, I'd be thin.

HAVE YOU SAID things like this before? It's time to get clear on this one. How many times have you actually been tied down and forced to eat? I'm guessing that no one has ever put food in your mouth against your will. I bet you've never been held at gunpoint and told to consume food, either.

Though these examples may sound ridiculous, they are no more absurd than blaming others for your weight problem. By trying to make someone else at fault you are refusing to take responsibility for your life. It works like this: if you can blame another person then taking action is also out of your control. In other words, you get to sit on your butt and eat rather than putting effort into recovering.

While it is possible, even likely, that many of us live with people who are less than supportive of our weight loss efforts, the choices we make are our own. And it's time we take responsibility for our own actions. If we choose to overeat then it is because we made that decision. No one else forced us to. We have the power to say no and we need to use it.

Rather than spending time blaming others for our emotional eating, we can use the time to practice setting boundaries. Begin by saying no every time someone offers you food. Don't explain why. Simply say, "No, thanks." That's it. No excuses. No long involved stories. Just two little words.

Chances are that after you have said no, you will feel guilty, scared, even angry. This is normal. It won't be fun to feel these things but it won't be forever. If you know that this will happen, then you can prepare for it.

For instance, if you've just refused food from someone you love, you may need to make a phone call to a supportive friend, write in your journal, or take a walk to deal with the feelings. Whatever you do, however, don't reach for food. Instead, simply let the feelings wash over you. If you're still having trouble with this, you'll read more on day fifty-one, "Brutal honesty about your feelings is necessary." For now, realize that you will not die from feeling uncomfortable emotions.

When you can stop blaming others for your weight problem you can begin taking responsibility for your actions and have the waistline you've always dreamed about.

30

Rachael Ray doesn't eat everything she cooks and neither should you.

Yes, Rachael Ray does love food. There's no doubt about that. Most of the chefs you see on Food Network, or peering from the covers of cookbooks, also love food. And most of them don't eat everything they cook.

Most of us have been raised to eat everything on our plates. Many of us feel driven to compulsively taste food as we are cooking or scrape the bottom of every bowl or pan. It's time to stop this. Understand that even food you eat during preparation counts in your daily intake. Tasting food while cooking is an easy way to lose track of what you are actually eating.

The best way to handle this problem is to have a "no eating while cooking" rule. Do not lick the spoon or taste the batter. Don't even think about slicing a piece off the roast or dipping your fork into the stuffing. Do not do it. Ever. For any reason. Stop this minute and never go back.

Yes, it may be scary to serve food that you haven't tasted. Yes, you may give your family or guests something that is less than perfect, and, yes, it is possible that someone may not like what you've prepared. Remember, your priority here is to stop eating emotionally. That is your number one priority without exception. Eating everything you cook, pleasing others with the food you've prepared, and living up to anyone else's expectations are not nearly as important as your need to change your patterns.

Yes, some people may not like your new behavior. They will have to learn to deal with it. This is your life you are fighting for. And as you fight, try to learn from Rachael Ray. She doesn't eat everything she cooks and neither should you.

31

Cooking shows can trigger a binge.

THEY SEEM SO innocent, even entertaining. Yet the truth is they can be deadly. Yes, I'm talking about cooking shows. You may think this is crazy. Take a moment to look at what's really going on when you are watching.

The entire point of these shows is to show you how to make exceptional meals and desserts. Many of these are items you would serve only on special occasions. Therefore, you are being presented with foods high in calories and fat. This being the case, you could say that this food is the superstar of all others. It's created to look unrealistically attractive and be idolized.

Much like the bodies of celebrities, the food presented in cooking programs is created to be perfect, without flaws. You are meant to drool over it and fantasize about it in the same way you do idyllic bodies. Of course, this is a major problem for emotional eaters. Even those shows that present healthy food can still trigger a binge. Healthy food or not, by watching cooking shows you are still using food to entertain yourself.

Watching cooking shows creates an even deeper emotional attachment to food. These programs foster a longing and excitement around food. As someone who is already emotionally attached to food, this is dangerous.

Many of us have made food such a part of our lives that we aren't even aware of the sneaky ways we have created to make our lives revolve around eating. How many cooking shows do you watch? How excited to do you feel when watching the meals being prepared?

Chances are that if you watch cooking shows you are very attached to them and angry about the advice in this entry. You are probably telling yourself something about having a right to watch whatever you want. You may even be considering putting this book down.

Before you do that, ask yourself how well the choices you have made so far are working for you. If your emotional eating wasn't a problem then you wouldn't have started reading this book in the first place, right?

Today, spend the day making a list of all the ways food is integrated into your life. Do you work at a grocery store? Are you a baker? Do you cook to relax? Are you the first to volunteer cookies for your children's school events? Is your idea of a hobby going out to dinner? Write them all down. This will be a crucial step in understanding how dangerous your emotional eating truly is.

32

For emotional eaters, cookbooks can be dangerous if not used correctly.

Yes, WHAT YOU read yesterday goes for cookbooks as well. In the same way that cooking shows glorify and create desire for food, cookbooks do the same. Think about the full-color pictures with perfectly created food. Don't they make you want to go out and get what's shown?

Not all cookbooks are dangerous. It's what you do with them that matters. Referencing a healthy recipe is quite different than reading a cookbook from cover to cover. Looking at a healthful eating book for ideas differs greatly from studying photos of desserts.

At one time in my life, I spent hours looking through cookbooks fantasizing about the food that was pictured. I read each recipe and tried to taste it in my mind. Of course, at the time I told myself that I was simply looking for a recipe.

I used other people as the excuse to look through the cookbooks but the truth is that it was always about me. Looking at the photos was a way for me to escape from my life. If I could fantasize about food then I didn't have to feel my feelings. I could distract myself.

The problem is that this distraction eventually led to eating large quantities of food. Many times I waited a little while before I would actually get the food that I was looking at but I always got it. And I always ate until I was sick.

So, yes, you do have the right to read anything you choose to. No one can tell you what to look at and what not to. You do need to be aware of the consequences should you choose to read cookbooks. It is your choice but it is also your responsibility. Today, make the choice that best supports the direction you'd like to go in. It's up to you.

33

*You don't need to make one more celebrity
richer by buying his/her diet book.*

IT'S THE LATEST greatest diet by the hottest celebrity out
there. Everybody's doing it. How can you not buy the
book? Why wouldn't you want to be on the cutting edge of
the diet world, especially with someone famous involved?

The answer is simple—there's no need for you to do any
more research. You have all of the answers you'll ever
need. The way to lose weight is very simple—eat moderate
amounts of nutritious foods and exercise.

There, now you have all of the information you need.
You never have to buy another book telling you what to eat
again. Purchasing these books is not an active step in
overcoming your emotional eating. Instead, it is a
distraction.

Think of it like this: you tell yourself that if you buy a
book then you are taking steps to losing weight when in
reality you are actually diverting your attention from taking an action that will directly result in making progress.
Rather than buying another celebrity diet book, prepare

a healthy meal or take a walk. These efforts will directly result in positive action.

Purchasing a book is what's known as a false action. It looks as if you are moving forward but you're not. It's an action distraction. Buying a book does not change your life unless you actually incorporate the information into your life through action.

To be clear, I am not suggesting that you never buy another book again. That would not only be stupid on my part but it is inaccurate. There are many wonderful books that can provide you with inspiration and information to change your life. You are reading one now.

The difference between books like this and diet books is that the latter "feed" your obsession with food. As someone who is reading this book, you have admitted that you are concerned about your emotional attachment to food. Therefore, buying books about food, even if they are disguised as celebrity diet books, is not a healthy action.

Make a decision today to stop buying celebrity diet books. Instead, focus on one action that will help you move forward in your healthful eating efforts. Attend a support group. Go to the gym. Write in your journal. Meditate. Do something healthy and you will see a greater profit in your own life, rather than someone else's.

34

*Most models and actresses eat too little
and exercise too much.*

THEIR BODIES ARE perfect. Their hair is stunning. They are dressed impeccably. There is no doubt that these are America's ideal women. So, why don't you look like that?

The answers are simple:

1. You don't have an army of stylists, coaches, chefs, and personal trainers.
2. You don't starve yourself nor do you have a trainer who can whip you into shape five hours a day.
3. Your life does not revolve around a career that forces you to treat your looks as your greatest commodity.

A major turning point for real women all over the world was when *Desperate Housewives* star Terri Hatcher removed her hair extensions and talked about her shoes that were a size too big at an awards ceremony last year. She told the audience that they had no idea what it takes to make her look as glamorous as she did that evening.

Terri's courage in getting honest about the extreme amount of effort that goes into making celebrities appear perfect is refreshing. Most of the time we only see the final results rather than the intense work that goes into creating these images. Several years ago, Jamie Lee Curtis posed without makeup or lights for a *More* magazine article. The photos that ran were not retouched. The fact that this event garnered so much publicity shows how unrealistic the images we see are.

Throughout the years, there have been many celebrities and models who have admitted to eating too little food and overexercising. Take a moment to consider that when you compare yourself to these women, you hold yourself up to a lifestyle that is unhealthy and even dangerous. By reading this book, you are committing to a healthy, positive lifestyle. It's time to acknowledge the contradictions, and put them to bed. Today, make the decision to stop comparing yourself or emulating unhealthy habits. Instead, stick to what works: eat healthy, sensible meals and exercise regularly. If you compare yourself to women whose careers depend upon unhealthy behaviors, you will only sabotage yourself.

35

There is no law that requires you to eat chocolate on holidays.

CHOCOLATE VALENTINE'S HEARTS. Chocolate Easter bunnies. Chocolate dreidels. Chocolate Santa Clauses. Even chocolate-covered strawberries for Independence Day. Every holiday seems to give us an excuse to eat chocolate.

Even if there isn't a specially designated chocolate item for a particular holiday, we still manage to get it in there with other chocolate treats such as brownies, ice cream, and cookies. Chocolate has become so pervasive that most of us can't even imagine a special occasion without it.

Well, now's the time to start. Chocolate and holidays are not legally bound together. It is not illegal for you to skip the chocolate during celebrations.

To actually go through with this you will need to rethink the way you look at special occasions. Each and every holiday has a particular meaning behind it and now is the time to explore this. Rather than looking at each holiday as an excuse to eat sweets, consider the reason for the gathering.

Whether it's Valentine's Day or the Fourth of July, we are celebrating a particular thing, not giving ourselves reasons to gorge on chocolate.

The denial we have about our eating habits spills into the holiday season. We tell ourselves that we will only eat chocolate on these specific days but the truth is that we begin eating days, even weeks, before *and* after the holiday.

Even more dangerous, we convince ourselves that the only way to truly celebrate is to eat special foods. When we do this we attach feelings of happiness to foods high in calories and fat. This creates a powerful emotional eating opportunity.

Instead of continuing this tradition, today make a decision to find one nonfood-related activity that you can do to celebrate each holiday that you observe. For instance, rather than eating candy on Valentine's Day you can choose instead to take a warm bath, make a fire in the fireplace, watch a special movie, go dancing, or even read a special book of poetry. It doesn't matter what it is that you do as long as you have a plan.

36

*Exercising is simply moving your body
once a day.*

MOVE YOUR BODY at least once a day doesn't only mean exercising. Instead, this can be as simple as parking your car at the end of the lot, taking the stairs instead of the elevator, or walking an extra lap around the mall. Anything that gets you to move a little more than normally will work.

Remember, this is not about thirty minutes of exercise (though this is a good idea). Moving your body means doing just a bit more activity than you did before. And, though an extra lap around the mall or walking up a few stairs may not seem worth the effort, it actually is.

Take small, deliberate steps each day. Most of us try to do one big task then get overwhelmed about continuing on a daily basis. Instead, true success comes from taking manageable daily actions.

Creating large tasks for yourself is a form of sabotage that feeds your denial. The bigger the chore is the less likely you will continue to do it in the long term. This is where moving your body fits in nicely. Simply do one thing daily, nothing big, just enough to make progress each day. Walk from the furthest parking spot. Fly a kite. Swim a few laps in the pool. Play a round of golf or a set of tennis.

So, get up right now and move your body. Take a few deep breaths, stretch your arms above your head. You can do this. It will only take a few seconds. And once you do it, you can feel secure in the knowledge that you are making progress every day.

37

Monday isn't the only day to begin a healthy eating plan.

I'll start on Monday.

Even better, I'll wait until the first Monday of the month to begin.

Or, better yet, I'll wait until the first Monday of the year.

The only problem is that I'll have all of that holiday food around. I better wait until the first of February. But, then again, Valentine's Day is in February. Maybe it would be better to wait for the first Monday in March but I will be preparing for Easter so maybe April or May would be better. . . .

EVEN THOUGH THIS may be an exaggeration, the truth is that most of us have postponed our weight loss efforts at one time or another. We have brainwashed ourselves to believe that we must wait for a certain day to begin eating in a healthy way.

This is not only untrue but it's actually a part of the denial system we create to allow ourselves to continue eating. If you don't have to begin until Monday then you can eat as much as possible before then.

Of course, what usually happens after this is that you've stocked up on so much food that you are unable to actually go through with it and start anew. Your system isn't prepared to instantly switch gears and neither are your emotions.

In fact, by waiting until Monday you have created an even deeper emotional attachment to food by making it your lost love. You tried to spend as much time as you could with food before you knew it wasn't going to be there anymore. Much like a separation in a relationship, you tried to love it as much as you possibly could before it left. And during your separation, you will be longing for it in the same way that you yearn for a lost love.

The best thing you can do right now if you haven't been doing so or if you've had some trouble is to begin a healthy eating plan this minute. It is normal in any program to experience difficulties or to be tempted. Don't let this overwhelm you. If you are having problems, you can begin again no matter what day it is. It doesn't matter what time it is or where you are. Just simply make a decision to begin eating in a healthful way. You may not be able to figure out exactly what this means for you at this minute but you can make a start now by choosing nutritious foods.

Don't put it off anymore. Don't wait for another Monday and certainly don't wait for another new year to begin. Now is the only moment in time you have. Don't waste it. Begin immediately!

38

There is no magical weight that will make your life perfect.

When I lose weight, I'll _____.

You FILL IN the blank. I'm sure you've thought about this many times in your life. Will you take a trip you've always wanted to? Or, will you be wearing a certain outfit or participating in a special activity? Whatever it is, you've probably been dreaming about it for quite a while.

Maybe it's not that you will *do* something. Instead, you may believe your life will be a certain way if you lose weight: perhaps you will finally have that relationship you've always dreamed of or maybe the most amazing job or the perfect place to live. Or, it could involve being accepted into a certain social club or organization.

When I weighed 328 pounds, I truly believed that if I could lose weight then my life would be perfect. Everyone would love me. I would have the perfect relationship and I would be completely happy in my job. I convinced myself that my life would be fulfilled when I saw that magical number on the scale.

I remember vividly the day I stepped on the scale to see that number. I expected everything would come to me that very day. I was devastated to realize that I still had the same old life I did before. I was desperately unhappy in my relationship at the time, my living situation was tenuous at best, and I didn't have the stability I wanted at my job. Somehow I believed that that magical number would solve every problem I had.

I didn't realize until later that I had set myself up to go back to my unhealthy eating habits. I had created a list of unrealistic expectations to ensure that I would be disappointed. Of course, disappointment would be the excuse I needed to overeat. Luckily, I realized what was happening before it was too late.

As you continue on in your program, it is important for you to be as realistic as possible. Rather than thinking about what will happen when you lose weight, concentrate on making today the best day that you can. All of these days will add up to an amazing life and gradually you will find yourself achieving your dreams, whether they be smaller goals or major life changes. Then, you will see that the number on the scale has nothing to do with it.

39

Your imperfections are a part of you.

HERE'S A SECRET—you're not perfect. And you never will be. You can try and try until you're exhausted but perfection just isn't possible. So, make a decision right here and now to begin accepting how you look. Rather than desperately searching to be perfect, accept yourself as you are. This will allow you to move forward.

To begin, make a decision to stop all criticism of yourself. You can do this in two ways. First, don't say mean things about yourself. For instance, if you call yourself stupid when you make a mistake or fat when you try a pair of pants on, stop it. Say instead, "I am human and humans will never be perfect."

The second thing you can do is to begin to say nice things to yourself. This may seem scary to you and you may not want to do it, but try to keep an open mind. Even if you start by telling yourself one nice thing each day, it will move you forward. You will notice that after a while you will criticize yourself less than you did before.

Please understand that it will not feel wonderful the first few times you are nice to yourself. It may even make you cry. You are so used to the criticism that the positive talk reminds you of exactly how mean you have been to yourself. At first, your mind feels unworthy of the nice things.

Even though accepting yourself as you are may feel uncomfortable, it is important that you continue. Don't give up and it will get easier. Before you know it, you will get used to hearing positive things about yourself. Eventually, you will even come to believe them. Today, find at least one nice thing to say about yourself. Maybe you have a great smile or pretty hair. Do you have an outgoing personality or can you tell a great joke? Whatever it is, you owe it to yourself to notice it.

40

It's what you do after a slip that matters most.

I'm such a failure.
I may as well just give up.
Why bother?

How MANY TIMES have you said these things to yourself after eating something that wasn't healthy? If you're like most of us, it happens more often than you would like.

The problem with this sort of thinking is that it allows you to continue overeating. You are human and slips in your healthy eating program may happen. It's what you do directly after them that matters most.

If you've over- or undereaten, understand that this doesn't have to continue. You have the power to stop right now, regroup, and get back to your healthy lifestyle. If you allow yourself to continue your damaging behavior, then you're contributing to the denial that tells you it's okay to hurt yourself and to keep doing so. You deserve better. Today, it's time for you to realize exactly how important it is for you to follow your food plan.

Right now, take a pen or pencil and make a list of all the benefits of eating healthfully. In other words, what do you get out of it? Is it more energy? A sense of accomplishment and self-esteem? A feeling of happiness? Better fitting clothes? A more positive attitude? Lower blood pressure? A healthy heart? A clear head? A more active lifestyle? More confidence?

Whatever it is, write it down. Now, look over the list and understand exactly what you have to lose by neglecting your new lifestyle. The only way to have those things you wrote on your list is to continue in this program. There is no other method. As much as you might wish it to be so, there is no other way to achieve good health, a clear head, a sense of accomplishment, and all of the other things on the list.

Now, take that list and put it on your refrigerator. If you do slip up, read your list and let it remind you to begin again immediately. The next time you feel yourself slipping from your healthy eating plan, take a look at your list and remind yourself of all you have to gain by sticking to the program.

41

Your ideal body may not be your reality.

I'VE ALWAYS WANTED to be a size 4. That's been my ideal for as long as I can remember. Every time I went on a diet I desperately tried to reach that goal. I dreamt endlessly about how wonderful my life would be if only I could wear size 4 clothing.

More than seventeen years later, I still have not reached that goal. With the damage that I have done to my body over the years, that is not a reality for me. Hanging skin on the lower half of my body and large calves make a size 4 just not possible considering where I've come from.

Does this mean that I should give up and eat everything in sight because I will never have my ideal body? Should I give up the good health, the energy, the clearheadedness, and self-esteem that my new way of life has given me simply because I won't reach my goal?

My guess is that you are sitting there thinking of course I shouldn't, that that would be crazy. Maybe so, but that's the way denial works—if I can't have exactly what I want then

I will give up on everything. This is why it's important for you to let go of your ideal body. Understand that you may or may not achieve what you've always hoped to. That doesn't matter right now.

Your job today is to simply concentrate on making this day a healthy one. Do not focus on the results that may or may not come over time. Instead, just worry about this one day. Each action that you take to live a healthy life will contribute to making your situation better.

Decide right now to let go of the ideal and begin to live the reality. Commit to follow through on one healthy action today and know that you are on your way to overcoming your emotional eating.

42

*If your hands are busy,
you won't reach for food.*

Have you ever thought about knitting? Painting? Taking photos? Golfing? Swimming? Woodworking? Or anything else that you can use your hands for?

If not, now is the time to develop a hobby or interest that involves being active. Watching television doesn't count. It's passive and can actually make you think about food more. Instead, find something that will involve action on your part.

For me, it's journal writing, working around my house, and reading. When I am actively involved in doing any of these activities, I am not thinking about food or eating. Instead, I am connecting with the experience at hand.

By finding a hobby now you will have an insurance plan during times when you are upset. Rather than turning to food to make you feel better during difficult times, you will have a healthy, nonfood-related outlet instead. You won't have to wonder what you should do. You will have a plan in place to get you through.

Journal writing is something that has saved my recovery on many occasions. Last night, I was devastated by the ending of a special relationship in my life. The pain was intense. I wanted to eat. The little voice inside my head told me that ice cream would make it better.

I knew that if I listened I would be in serious trouble. I also realized that I needed to distract myself from these thoughts. I reached for a pen and my journal and began writing. And, as it always has before, it worked to calm me down and banish my food thoughts.

Today, think about what kind of a hobby you may want to pursue. It doesn't have to be anything big. It can be tending to flowers or plants, coloring with crayons, reading mysteries, or writing a novel, anything that will keep your hands busy and your mind engaged. It doesn't matter what it is as long as you like it and can do it when you need to.

43

You can't handle your feelings alone.

THE LONELINESS I feel wells up inside of me. Tears fall and I begin to sob uncontrollably from deep within a place I hoped never to visit again. It is the place where all of my pain lives. And it is overwhelming.

Though I try hard to ignore it, the voice grows stronger. It shouts inside of my head trying desperately to convince me that what it says is true; that food will make all of my pain go away; and that my life will be better if only I reach for ice cream.

No matter how many years of recovery I have, I can't handle this pain alone. I need help to get through. I wish I didn't and it makes me angry that I do but it is a reality of my life. I need help.

At this point, I know that I have a choice. I can either reach for the ice cream or I can reach out to others who understand. One will cause further devastation. The other, though unfamiliar and frightening, will allow me to continue following my program. With tears in my eyes,

I pick up the phone and begin to talk to my friend. The thoughts of ice cream slowly disappear. . . .

It is my hope that after reading this you will realize how important it is not only to have friends but to have people who are like you in your life. To find them, you can join a support group such as Overeaters Anonymous, a private eating disorders group, or a healthy eating group.

What matters most is that you have people in your life who understand your struggles with food. These people don't have to be your best friends or take up residence at your house. You just have to be able to contact them when you want to stray from your program.

Today, make an attempt to research one of these groups. Go online and search for a support group for people who struggle with food or look for an Overeaters Anonymous meeting in your area (www.overeatersanonymous.org) or contact a local counseling center to ask what they offer. Local libraries, community centers, and places of worship often have listings for support groups. Take one step to meet people like you and it will save your life someday soon. It did mine.

44

No one can lose weight for you.

I don't want to do this. Maybe you can cook and shop for me. After all, it's your fault that I'm having so many problems with food. You're such a good cook and you bring all of this food into the house. If you didn't bring that into the house then I wouldn't eat it.

How many times have you wished someone could lose weight for you? It may be that you've never thought of it this directly but chances are that the thought has crossed your mind in one way or another.

The biggest clue to when this is happening is that you are blaming others for your eating: *He did this to me. She isn't doing what I want her to. If only she would* _____ *(fill in the blank), I would stop eating.* Phrases such as these are clues to what's really going on in your mind.

You're giving your power away to someone else. If they were different, then you would be. Unfortunately, it doesn't work this way. In order to overcome your emotional eating you will need to take full responsibility for your actions and choices.

To begin, you will need to let go of the idea that it is someone else's job to lose weight for you. You will need to take charge of your own eating plan. This means that it is your sole responsibility to shop for the food you need, to prepare the meals you eat, and to manage your feelings.

While the first two seem logical it's the third that needs more explanation. One of the most subtle ways that we try to get others to lose weight for us is by expecting them to make our lives better that will, in turn, make us feel happier. This is not only dangerous to your healthy eating, it is unfair to others.

No one can make you feel better but you. Even though you may be happy in a relationship with someone else, this person cannot make you feel happy. Your unique experience in the relationship is what causes the good feelings. What you feel good about may not be the same for someone else.

You are a complex person whose reactions and feelings are based on your own personal growing experiencing. There is no one else out there like you therefore no one else can make your feelings better or lose weight for you.

Today, take some time to get to know this person who you will be with for the rest of your life—yourself. What do you like to do? When do you feel happy? Sad? Excited? Looking deeper into these things will help you to understand yourself better and to take responsibility for every area of your life.

45

Not all magazines send negative body image messages.

W<small>HY WOULD</small> I suggest that you read a glossy magazine when I've written extensively about the dangers of the unrealistic images they promote? It's actually quite simple. Reading a fitness magazine, if done in a healthy way, can actually motivate you.

Before you reach for the magazine take a few seconds to understand that you are not trying to look like the celebrities and models featured in the pages. If you can, try to ignore the photos, concentrating instead on the text and what you can learn from it. For instance, is there a story about a workout or a new way to stick with an exercise program? These types of articles can go a long way in keeping you committed to your new lifestyle.

Another thing to avoid is stories offering new diets and weight loss suggestions. Even though you may be tempted to look at the next greatest diet, take a second to go back a few entries and reread entry 11. The perfect diet doesn't exist.

Ideally, you should try to find a fitness magazine that concentrates on exercise more than eating habits or cooking suggestions. If there is too much emphasis on food and weight loss then you will defeat the original purpose of reading the magazine—to get motivated.

So, go ahead and grab a fitness magazine. Read the stories that will motivate you and make a decision to follow at least one of the suggestions. As you do so, remember you are reading these magazines to help your body not soothe your emotions. Rather than using the images in these magazines to harm your body image, you can make a decision to change the way you look at them. It's in your hands.

46

You're not the only one hurt by your emotional eating.

I'M NOT HURTING *anyone by overeating.* Eighteen years ago, I truly believed these words. Today, I know differently.

When I weighed over 300 pounds, I was so desperately miserable that I didn't know what my loved ones were experiencing. Both of my parents worried about my health. My sister was teased viciously for having a fat sibling. And those few people who did spend time with me were ostracized for doing so.

Every day the people in my life were forced to deal with my sadness, depression, and anger. And though I tried not to, I regularly took my frustration out on those around me. In short, I was miserable to be around yet I didn't know it.

Is it possible that this is happening in your life? For the past forty-five days you have learned a lot about yourself and your eating habits. Up until this point, the focus has been on you. Today, it's time to think about the other people in your life.

Has anyone ever told you that they are worried about your over- or undereating? Have you ever pushed someone away so that you could be alone to eat? Has your anger with yourself spilled over into other areas of your life or been used as a weapon to keep people away? Or, have you given up and pulled away from everyone?

These are only a few of the ways that your eating patterns can affect others. You probably have your own habits outside of those mentioned above. Think about all areas of your life. Do you stifle your career so that you have more time to be with food? Is your living space all that you want it to be or do you simply ignore it so you have time to eat? Are your spending habits out of control because you're buying so much food?

Today, take some time to write about the ways that your eating impacts other people in your life. Don't use this list to beat yourself up. Instead, use this list to motivate you to make things better. You deserve to have a full and healthy life, not just for yourself but for your loved ones as well.

47

You can accept your body
with childlike wonder.

SNAP YOUR FINGERS. Clap your hands. Hold your breath. Wiggle your toes. Move your legs. And reach your arms up into the air.

How does that feel? Are you grateful that you can do these things? Do you grow impatient with the movements? Are you unhappy about the way you felt? Do you criticize your body?

Even if you aren't criticizing your body this time, you probably have before. Today is your chance to change that. To begin, take a moment to do the exercises in the first paragraph again. As you do them, think about how wonderful it is that your fingers can make a snapping noise. Revel in the fact that your hands can applaud. Enjoy the feeling of your toes moving and your arms reaching up into the air.

Focus on the wonder of your movements. Try to think of yourself as a child. Small children are amazed when they learn to snap their fingers or clap their hands. They are filled with excitement by their accomplishments. Babies don't criticize the size of their hips or legs. They don't have the capacity to judge their bodies. They only take joy in their movements and do not find fault with their size.

Repeating this exercise every morning will help remind you of the power you hold. You may also want to write down a list of the things your body can accomplish. The next time you begin to criticize your body, refer to this list and take joy in your abilities. After all, you are a biological miracle.

48

No one will die if you say no to dessert.

OKAY, DEATH MAY sound a bit dramatic. But how many times do you tell yourself that you must eat dessert because someone worked hard for it? That your mom will feel bad if you don't eat the brownies she made or that your friend will get angry if you don't devour the expensive pastry she bought? And, how often do you convince yourself that the other person's well-being depends on you eating it?

My guess is that you've done this at least once. It's time to think about the reasoning here: If you can convince yourself that you must eat the dessert in order to make your mother or your friend feel good, then the stakes become higher.

As emotional eaters, we are all too familiar with feelings of pain. Chances are that we feel hurt or sad on a regular basis, perhaps even more so than those who don't use food the way we do. While being familiar with this kind of pain can provide us with deeper levels of compassion, it can also feed the denial that fuels our emotional eating.

When we feel "forced" to eat food someone has pre-pared, we tell ourselves that we are protecting others from the intense pain we regularly feel. At first glance, this seems noble. Unfortunately, this isn't the case.

The truth is that we are using "protecting other people's feelings" as an excuse to eat foods that aren't good for us.

What someone else feels is not your responsibility. Each person is different and his or her reactions are made up of their personal experiences and feelings. You do not have the power to make anyone feel anything. Their feelings are based on their own life's events.

You are not so powerful that you get to decide how other people will feel. You don't have any say about what others think. The only person who you can control is yourself. Today, stop trying to convince yourself that eating dessert is a life and death matter. No one will die if you don't eat dessert. You are not responsible for anyone else's feelings. Repeat that over and over to yourself until you truly believe this healthy truth.

49

The food pyramid was created for a reason (and it's not to torment you).

Yes, we've all heard the criticisms about the food pyramid. To be sure, there are problems with it—even the newly revised one—especially for those physically addicted to sugar and flour. There are, however, some suggestions worth thinking about.

Did you notice that there isn't a candy or ice cream section on either pyramid? There are no potato chips or corn chips. There isn't a place for cupcakes or doughnuts. Cookies and whipped cream aren't included, either. There are reasons for these exclusions: The foods mentioned above are not nutritionally necessary.

Instead, the USDA suggests that adults eat 2½ cups of vegetables and 2 cups of fruit daily. Look at your own eating patterns. Think about how close you come to that amount. When is the last time you ate 2½ cups of vegetables and 2 cups of fruit in one day?

Hopefully, you've been trying to incorporate more fruits and vegetables into your daily meals since beginning this program. If not, why not? Perhaps you tell yourself that you don't like vegetables or fruit. Maybe you say that you don't have time to cook. But, how true are either of these things?

How many vegetables have you actually tried? Are you operating under an outdated belief from your childhood about the taste? Have you tried to prepare the fruits or vegetables in different ways or are you just content to rely on the memory of what you think you know?

Today is the day for you to make changes. Go to the grocery store and find at least three different types of vegetables and fruits you are willing to try. Then, go to the spice aisle and select several spices and/or sauces that you can use in preparation. Try to stick to low-fat sauces such as salsa, tomato sauce, or mustard.

Now, make a commitment to experiment with at least one new vegetable dish at dinner each day. Or, you may even choose to lightly steam or eat the vegetables raw. And don't stick to just vegetables, either. Look for fruits that you haven't tried and incorporate them into your meal as well. Understand that you may have something you don't like. That's okay. The important thing is that you are willing to try different things. If none of these things appeal to you then try more and keep trying until you find something you do like. And remember, strawberry ice cream doesn't count as a fruit.

50

Food manufacturers weren't joking when they outlined serving sizes.

Is half a cup really the serving size for oatmeal? Do people really eat that amount? Or, how about three ounces of meat for females and four for males? When's the last time these people went to a restaurant? Portions there are usually more than triple those amounts. Those serving sizes can't be right.

WHEN IS THE last time you ate the suggested portion outlined on a food package? Can you remember when you even read these guidelines?

Yesterday, you read that the food pyramid was created for a reason. The serving sizes on packages were also established as realistic guidelines for healthful eating.

For many of us, following these suggestions brings up a lot of emotion. At first, we feel angry. Who has the right to tell us what to eat? Then, we begin to feel fear. If we eat the recommended amounts then we are afraid we will be hungry. Perhaps there is even some sadness. Why do we have to be limited so while others are able to manage their eating?

Each individual is different, therefore your feelings may not follow this exact pattern. But as an emotional eater, it is inevitable that you will have strong feelings about being asked to limit your food intake. Food has served as your solace, best friend, even escape for years. Being asked to place limits on these "comfort zones" can be a frightening prospect.

The challenge here is to find another way to comfort yourself. Many have been outlined over the past forty-nine days (read, write, take a bath, take a walk, etc.). You will need to find the ones that work for you. By nurturing yourself in other ways, you begin to put food in its proper place—as a means of nourishing yourself, not as a means of emotional solace.

Today, make it a point to notice the serving sizes on the items you are eating. Make an attempt to follow the suggestions. Then, jot down your feelings about doing this. Are you angry? Sad? Upset? Scared? Remember, you can't choose your feelings but you do have a choice about your actions. Today, choose to take another step toward eating realistic portions.

51

*It is best to decide what to eat
when you are full.*

MOST OF US don't plan our meals. Instead we reach for whatever we can find when we're hungry. If it happens to be at a mealtime then we may choose to call it breakfast, lunch, or dinner. If not, we eat it anyway.

For some of us, mealtime is one never-ending period during the entire day. There is no set eating time or beginning and ending to the meals. We graze throughout the whole day never taking even a second to plan.

For those of us with children or families, perhaps we make an attempt to serve three meals during the day and even put some effort into planning them. Our problem appears to be more contained. After all, we don't eat much at mealtime so why do we have this problem? It's what we are eating between these meals or at night when we are alone that causes us difficulties.

In both cases, the importance of planning healthy meals must not be underestimated. Yes, I said *planning*. I can hear your protests. Who wants to plan? Why shouldn't you eat whatever you want when you want?

The truth is that you do have every right to eat anything at any time. But the question to ask yourself is how well has that been working for you? Are your eating patterns the way you want them to be? Is your life happy? Do you feel peaceful? Is your body a size you're comfortable with? In short, is this what you want for yourself?

My guess is that you've answered no to many of the above questions. If you are not happy with your life then the only solution is to try doing things differently. It's just that simple. There is no other way to change.

Today, after you finish reading, plan three meals for yourself. Begin with breakfast. Don't allow yourself any excuses about not being able to eat in the morning. Remember, you have made a decision to do things differently. Give it a try. I've outlined a basic plan below, but you may want to consult a nutritionist or registered dietician to develop a more personalized healthy eating plan. For breakfast, plan to eat about a cup or one piece of fruit, a protein such as half of a cup of nonfat, plain yogurt, a quarter of a cup of cottage cheese, two egg whites, or a quarter of a cup of ricotta cheese, whole grain cereal without sugar or flour, and a cup of non- or lowfat milk. Look at the serving sizes on the containers to determine the amount for the cereal.

Next, plan to eat lunch four to five hours after breakfast. Include three ounces of a lowfat protein such as chicken, fish, turkey, or tofu, two cups of vegetables such as lettuce, tomatoes, green beans, broccoli, cauliflower, mushrooms, a starch such as chickpeas, kidney beans, barley, or black beans, and a fruit.

Dinner, which should be four or five hours after lunch, should be similar to lunch without the fruit and adding a fat such as butter or margarine. You may or may not want to include an evening snack four hours after dinner. This should include a fruit, a protein such as nonfat yogurt, and a cereal.

Now it's up to you. Take a few minutes to plan out one day of meals and make a decision not to eat anything else no matter what happens. After all, the only thing you have to lose is your emotional dependence on food. Isn't that a weight off your mind and body?

52

*Brutal honesty about your feelings
won't hurt anyone.*

Now THAT YOU are several days past the halfway point, you are probably experiencing many different feelings. You may feel glad to know that you're not alone, angry that you have this problem, sad that there is no magic cure, or excited about the possibilities a new life can offer.

No matter what you are feeling, the most important thing is for you to be honest. Chances are that up until now you have had difficulty expressing your feelings and sometimes even identifying them. You may have spent a lifetime denying or ignoring what you are feeling.

To deal with your emotional eating you will need to really think about your feelings. You will have to be able to identify them so that you can understand where your urge to over- or undereat comes from.

To begin, right now take a deep breath and think about how you are feeling. If you're like I was, you may not even know how to name your feelings. At first, I needed to break my feelings down into four simple words. I offer these to you right now: sad, mad, glad, and scared.

If you're unsure, chances are that one of these four will help you to name it. Though there are many other emotions that stem from these, this is a good start.

While you are doing this, try not to confuse feelings with thoughts. For example, saying, "I feel rejected" does not express a true feeling. Being rejected is a state of mind not a feeling. Instead, try to think about what's beneath the thought. You may be feeling sad, mad, scared, even glad depending on the situation.

Once you can learn to acknowledge your true emotions, this honesty will flow into all areas of your life—including your eating habits. Today, make a decision to learn the healthy truth about brutal honesty. And remember, being honest is the kindest thing you can do for yourself and those around you.

53

*Wearing big clothes only makes you
look bigger.*

THOUGH MOST OF us have been conditioned from
childhood to wear tentlike shirts to make us appear thinner, the result is actually the opposite. Wearing a big shirt
actually adds to your size. Still not sure? Think about it
for a second.

Compare a tight-fitting shirt to a tent shirt. Which
one takes up less space? It's not the tentlike shirt, is it?
This being so, why would you think that wearing more
material on your body would make you look thinner?

If this is true then wouldn't tucking your shirt in make
you look thinner? Rather than appearing to be one large,
shapeless blob with a tentlike shirt, you can choose to
tuck in your shirt. This would, at the very least, give you
a nice figure instead.

After reading this, you may be horrified. You are probably telling yourself that there is no way you are ever going
to tuck in your shirt. But before making that decision, finish reading the rest of this.

You need to be willing to try to put years of conditioning behind you. You can stop believing that only thin people are allowed to tuck in their shirts. It may feel uncomfortable but it's important to give yourself a chance to get used to it. Since this may be the first time you've ever done this, it is only natural that it would feel odd. Become familiar with how it feels to have your shirt tucked in. Look in the mirror a few times. Take pictures and study them. Is there a difference? Be honest.

The first time I tucked in my shirt, I thought I was going to die. I was sure that everyone was looking at my enormous stomach. I had been very careful my whole life to wear tight jeans with enormous shirts in an attempt to hide my fat. But my therapist had suggested I give it a try.

As I left my room, my heart was pounding and I felt sick. I didn't want to be seen in public. All I wanted to do was hide. I trusted my therapist so I decided to give it a try, even though I was repulsed by the idea.

Walking out of my room, my friend said, "You're tucking in your shirt now."

"Yes," I said, carefully placing my arms across my stomach to cover my fat.

"You look really good," she smiled. "This way, you have a shape. With those big shirts, you didn't have a waist. They made you look heavier."

Even though I didn't believe her, I was at least open to the possibility that she was telling the truth. After a few similar comments from others, I was able to look in the mirror and see that I truly did look better. It took me longer to get over my feelings of self-consciousness, but they did eventually disappear.

Today I can wear my shirt tucked in and know that it really is more flattering than wearing a tentlike shirt. I no longer have to hide my shape underneath an enormous shirt. And I learned all of this because I was willing to suffer through a little discomfort. Today, will you do the same?

54

Weighing yourself too often puts your
emotions on the scale.

HOW MANY TIMES a week or month do you step on the scale? Are you one of those weigh-yourself-every-day people? Is the scale part of your morning routine?

If so, it may be time to reconsider your actions. First, think about what stepping on the scale every morning does to your emotional state. If the numbers are to your liking then you feel happy; if they're not then your whole day is ruined. Either way, your emotions are directly connected to the numbers on the scale and not your inner self.

Ideally, we would be able to completely separate our emotions from our body size but this takes time. One of the ways we can help overcome our emotional reliance on food is to make a decision to weigh ourselves only once a month.

If weighing yourself only once a month seems extreme, it may be a good idea for you to think about the reasons for this. Why is getting on the scale every day so important to you? Is it a way to justify eating whatever you want or is it a means to punish yourself?

For me, it was both. If I lost weight then somewhere in the back of my mind was the idea that I could eat more. Of course, I got a temporary high from the lower numbers but I also used them to justify overeating. If I gained weight, I then told myself how weak and pathetic I was and proceeded to eat high calorie foods to make myself feel better. Whatever the number on the scale, the end result was always the same: I ate.

Now, instead of putting myself in that position, I weigh myself only once a month. And even though it was difficult to stay off the scale in the beginning, I now experience a freedom that I didn't know was possible. My emotional state is no longer centered on the scale. Instead, I can live a life based on my true feelings, not ones determined by my weight.

Why not give it a try? Today, make a decision not to step on the scale. Choose a date that you'll remember. For me, it's the 14th of every month, which is the day I was released from treatment. Then, make a commitment to only weigh yourself on that day every month. And enjoy the freedom!

55

Food doesn't have to be on every guest list.

LET'S HAVE LUNCH. Or, better yet, how about dinner? We can have a working breakfast or even a celebration dessert.

Have you ever realized exactly how many events revolve around food? Even people who aren't emotional eaters find it hard to imagine a gathering without food. But, as an emotional eater, there are more considerations than you may be willing to acknowledge.

Think about how you feel when you are in social situations. Are you anxious? Do you feel self-conscious? Awkward? Shy? Unable to relate to others? Do you spend a great deal of time trying to please others without thinking about what you want or need?

Chances are that you've answered yes to at least one of the questions above. Now, think about the fact that food is present. As an emotional eater, you have learned to use food to deal with your feelings. If you are at a social event that is bringing up strong emotions then your first thoughts will turn to food.

You may even find yourself eating more than ever at these events. Or, if you are prone to secretive eating as many of us are then you may either eat a lot before or after. Either way, the result is the same—you are using food to deal with your feelings about being social.

Today, make a decision to host a gathering that doesn't involve food. It doesn't have to be a big party. It can be an informal get-together with a friend. Find an activity that does not include eating. Perhaps you can take a walk together, go to a flea market or antique show, attend a lecture, go to a yoga class, plant some flowers, or volunteer.

In the future, you can plan larger events, parties, and celebrations that don't revolve around food. For instance, how about a bowling or hiking party? Or a craft gathering? It doesn't matter what you do just that you are willing to think about having a food-free event. It may be tricky at first but after a few times you won't even regret leaving food off of the guest list.

56

Jokes about your body size are not funny.

I HATE COMEDIANS. Okay, maybe that's a bit strong. A better way to say it is that I don't find any humor whatsoever in fat jokes. They are mean and vicious. As an overweight child, I was the brunt of not only jokes but cruel teasing that often left me fearful for my life.

Maybe you think that if you are the first one to joke about your body size then no one else will. Perhaps there is some truth in this but consider the price you pay. By telling these jokes you are sending yourself the message that you are not good enough. Even in jest, this hurts your already fragile self-esteem. And when you are hurt, where do you turn? To food?

One of the most effective ways to help end emotional eating is to become aware of the things you say about yourself to others. Are you constantly making sarcastic remarks about yourself, your capabilities, or your actions? Do you regularly insult or downplay your accomplishments?

If so, you can make a concerted effort to change the way you talk about yourself. After becoming aware of your words, you can begin to make different choices. For instance, if you constantly joke about how many rolls of fat you have, you can simply make a decision not to mention this. If you are tempted, pull out the list you made on day twenty-two and reread it.

As you go through your day today, become aware of the words you say about yourself. Then, make steps to turn them into positive statements all the while knowing that fat jokes aren't funny or harmless, especially when you make them about yourself.

57

No amount of makeup can hide puffiness in your face.

If I can just find the perfect makeup then maybe no one will notice the rest of my body.

If my lashes are long enough then people will look into my eyes and not at the rest of me.

THOUGHTS LIKE THESE are common for emotional eaters. Concentrating on things that seem easier is less overwhelming. Going out and buying makeup appears to be a way to improve our looks or take care of ourselves yet in reality it distracts us from the real problem—our emotional eating.

There is no amount of makeup that will hide the puffiness in your face that comes from overeating. You can't cover up the deep misery of abusing yourself. Making yourself look good on the outside does not truly cover up the reason you are unhappy.

Searching for the perfect eye shadow or sweater is a distraction from dealing with the issues that surround our emotional eating. We can get so caught up in trying to hunt down the one thing that we think will make us feel better that we fail to deal with our real pain.

Today, rather than putting your efforts into your external appearance, think about your emotional state. As you are reading this what feelings are coming up? Are you sad, mad, glad, or scared? Can you see the truth in this entry or do you want to pretend that you never read it? Do you want to run away from this or are you ready to face your feelings and look inside?

There are no right or wrong answers. The important thing here is that you connect with your emotions. By taking some time to think about your feelings you are taking an important step. If you stop trying to cover up your emotional eating your real beauty will shine through.

58

Searching for the magic pill will keep you from recovering.

H OW MANY TIMES have you wished for a magic pill that would make you lose weight overnight? Judging from the soaring sales of diet pills, you're not alone. Before they were recalled, prescription diet pills Redux and Phen/Fen were the biggest selling drugs of their time. They sold at a rate unequaled by most drugs on the market today.

What's important to remember, however, is that these pills were later proven to be dangerous, even deadly. While pills may benefit a few people, there are risks for many.

Even more important, we need to recognize the truth here: What you are looking for is a pill that will allow you to lose weight while eating whatever you want. Isn't that right? Well, remember, there is no such pill. With any weight-loss medication, you must still maintain a healthy diet and exercise regularly. This being so, why would you risk your life by taking medication that you really don't need?

Since the side effects of diet pills are so dangerous, you cannot keep taking them forever. What happens when you stop? In most cases, you gain the weight back almost instantly. Ultimately, the only people who benefit from diet pills are drug manufacturers.

Rather than searching so hard for a magic cure to make you thin, you need to instead concentrate on taking consistent, healthy actions on a daily basis. If you put as much energy into eating healthfully and exercising regularly as you do into fantasizing or searching for a magic cure, you would have already lost the weight you wanted to!

It's time to give up the fantasy of eating whatever you want, whenever you want. This doesn't work. Now you need to admit that pills aren't the answer and move on.

Today is the day that you have a chance to change the way you've been looking at your dieting career. Rather than continuing to search for that perfect pill that will make you lose weight, it's time to admit how dangerous and counterproductive diet pills are, and recognize that this "perfect pill" method does not exist. It's time to embrace the healthy truth, rather than live in a world of weight-loss fantasies.

59

Dieting is not a competitive sport.

LOSING WEIGHT IS not a contest. There is no finish line and no winner. You will not be given a prize for losing weight faster than your significant other, best friend, sister, brother, or parent. Everyone loses weight at a different pace.

Even though it is natural to feel jealous when someone else loses weight faster than you, you don't have to let these feelings sabotage your efforts. For many of us, someone else's success becomes an excuse to reach for food. We tell ourselves that we will never be as good as he or she is so why even bother?

By doing this, you are giving yourself a reason to use food as a means of soothing your emotions. You have put yourself in the victim mode. You tell yourself that you aren't good enough so you may as well give up. Convenient, isn't it?

Realize that comparing yourself to anyone for any reason is always going to make someone the loser. You're either going to feel better than the person you've chosen or worse. Either way, someone comes out on the short end.

Even though you are conditioned to be competitive in your work life, you do not have to let this carry over into your personal care. You can simply acknowledge any feelings you may have about someone else's success then confirm your commitment to your own health.

You can also make a decision to use the person's weight-loss success to your own benefit. If this person has used healthy methods perhaps she can serve as an example of what you can accomplish. Or, if the weight-loss methods are unhealthy, you can learn from her experience by reminding yourself that lasting changes take time.

Today, you can take joy in the fact that you are moving forward in your own healthy eating program. You do not have to compare yourself to anyone else. Someone else's success has nothing to do with you. You are not a failure because they have succeeded. You can make progress at your own pace and realize that you are okay no matter what anyone else is doing.

60

Hunger pains won't kill you.

IT'S YOUR BIGGEST fear. You do whatever it takes to avoid feeling it. Maybe you don't even know what it feels like. It's the thing you've avoided all of your life: feeling hungry.

Some of us truly believe that we will die if we feel hungry. Depending on when we grew up, we may have been conditioned to deeply fear hunger. If you grew up during the Depression or World Wars when food was scarce and/or rationed, you have developed an attitude of scarcity. Sometimes this attitude is passed down through several generations so even if you are younger you may still experience feelings of scarcity.

If you doubt that this "scarcity mentality" is present today, think about the growing popularity of warehouse stores where food is purchased in large quantities. If you're a member of one of these, look around at the overflowing carts.

All of this translates into one big fear: that we will somehow starve to death. In most cases, today in our country this is not a valid fear. Even the most financially challenged of us have governmental aid available. Food drives are held regularly and shelters are available for those needing help. No matter what happens in your life, you will have enough food. It is not necessary for you to overcompensate.

Today, you can realize that you do not have to act out your fear of feeling hunger by hoarding and bingeing. In truth, if you are eating sensible meals then you should begin to feel hungry around mealtime. This is normal and you won't die. You just simply need to stick with your program and understand that hunger is a normal part of life—not a death sentence.

61

Having only one size of clothing in your closet keeps you honest.

THERE'S THE SKINNY clothes. Then, the really skinny clothes. And, of course, the fat clothes and the really fat clothes.

Many of our closets are filled with outfits that we may wear "someday," outfits that we can't bear to part with. At first, you may think that your closet has nothing to do with the emotional health of your eating habits. Yet, think about it. How do you feel when you open the door to your closet in the morning? Do you feel ashamed that you can't fit into some of your clothes or that you are wearing the largest sizes you have?

Whatever your experience is, it's time to look at it. Perhaps you have been living with the idea that having various sizes in your closet doesn't cause you emotional pain. Maybe you've never thought about the consequences. Either way, today make a decision to create a nurturing environment.

To begin, take everything out of the closet. I know. I know. I can hear the groans but why not give it a try? What do you have to lose? If time doesn't allow you to do this today then make a date in the next day or two to do this. Write it on your calendar the same way you would a doctor or dentist appointment. And stick to it. Assemble boxes or bags to use for the clothing you will be discarding. Then, go on to tomorrow's entry so you will have something to do today.

After you have taken everything out of your closet, take some time to examine all of the clothing you have. Inventory each item. In order for it to go back into the closet, it must pass three tests: It must fit properly. It must feel comfortable. You must love it. While this may severely limit the number of clothes you have, chances are that if you're honest you really are wearing only a small portion of everything in your closet anyway.

Before you put things back you may want to consider developing a plan to paint the closet or buy matching hangers or perhaps even put up inspirational sayings or photos. The goal here is to make going into your closet a pleasant experience. As emotional eaters, we have made a lifetime out of feeling negatively about our bodies. Our clothing is an extension of this as is our closet.

For many of us, our closets are frightening reminders of our entire emotional eating history. By creating a pleasant environment, you are giving yourself a gift, reminding yourself of your commitment to healthy eating and your new way of life. Every morning when you wake up you will feel nurtured and inspired when dressing. You deserve this so take some time to be nice to yourself.

62

Your too-small bathing suit is holding you captive.

▬

It sits there in your drawer. You look at it almost daily thinking how much you'd like to wear it again. And you criticize yourself for the weakness and lack of willpower that prevents you from being able to. It's the most feared item of the summer season: the bathing suit.

No matter what your feelings are about the words bathing suit, and whether or not you actually have one in your drawer, my message for you is the same: It's time to stop beating yourself up for not being able to wear it. Much like spending a lot of your energy pursuing the perfect body, trying to make yourself fit into a too-small bathing suit only serves to make you feel inadequate and unworthy.

And when we fall short of our goals, then the first place we turn is to the refrigerator. Trying to have the perfect body is actually an excuse to make ourselves feel badly and overeat. If you are following a healthy eating plan, you will reach a healthy body size. You may never be perfect but you will be a whole lot healthier and happier.

Today is the day that you let go of the idea of being able to wear that too-small bathing suit. If you have one, throw it away, burn it, or rip it up. You are no longer bound by unrealistic images of beauty. You do not have to beat yourself up. You can stop that right now. You may even want to buy a new bathing suit that fits properly.

As you strive to follow a healthy eating plan, be gentle and accepting of yourself. Do not abuse yourself for what you are not today. This is the only day you have. And if you are using the inability to wear a too-small bathing suit to beat yourself up then you need to stop. Get rid of the bathing suit and free yourself from the captivity of feeling bad!

63

You do deserve an occasional reward.

YOU'RE NOW MORE than two-thirds of the way through this program. If you've been consistently reading the entries and completing the activities you've learned a lot. You are now aware of many new things and probably noticing an improvement in your eating habits.

Now, it's time to treat yourself. Even if you haven't done every exercise yet or your eating habits aren't quite where you'd like them to be, you have still made important progress in overcoming your emotional eating. Simply picking up this book and reading parts of it has provided you with more information than you had before. And that deserves to be rewarded.

If you're like most food addicts or emotional eaters then your first thoughts involve food. This is to be expected. For years, you have been trained to think about food as a means to reward yourself. Today is the day that you begin to look at things differently.

Even though rewarding yourself is a positive thing, you may be experiencing some resistance or fear. Perhaps you're unsure how to reward yourself. Again, this is to be expected. For a good portion of your life, you have not even considered rewarding yourself unless food was involved. Or, maybe you felt as if you didn't deserve to be rewarded.

Though all of this is understandable, it is important for you to follow through and do something nice for yourself. You may not even know what that is yet but taking the time to figure it out is vital to overcoming your emotional eating.

This may be the first time you have rewarded yourself with anything other than food. By doing this, you will begin to experience good feelings from something that doesn't involve eating. This will give you a base upon which to build. And even if it doesn't feel good at first, keep trying until it does. It will when you are ready.

Be gentle with yourself and find something you enjoy. Try a massage. Get a manicure. Buy a new outfit. Treat yourself to a movie or show. Go to a concert. Take a hike in a special place. Go to an amusement park. Visit a museum. Go to an antiques store or a flea market. Find what works for you. Try different things. Make it a monthly ritual to reward yourself. You deserve it!

64

Hurting yourself even in subtle ways affects your eating.

Yᴏᴜ ᴋɴᴏᴡ ʏᴏᴜ hurt yourself with food. You are aware that eating items high in calories and fats is dangerous to your body. You understand that not exercising is harmful and you are very clear that using food to cope rather than expressing your emotions causes all sorts of physical ailments.

What you may not know are the subtle ways you hurt yourself. These are much more difficult to notice but they are just as damaging and, most times, result in emotional eating. For instance, how many times have you denied yourself basic things such as going to the bathroom when you have to, resting when you're tired, or adjusting the temperature when you're hot or cold?

Take a second right now to think about how your body feels. Are you hot or cold? Is the chair you're sitting in comfortable? If you are standing, does that feel good? How does your body feel? Is your back sore? Do your feet hurt? Are you hungry or overly full? Is there anything else going on physically?

How about your emotional state? Are you angry about reading this? Do you feel relieved? Are you happy? Or, do you feel overwhelmed? If you're unsure, as many emotional eaters are, remember the four basic feelings: sad, mad, glad, scared. Do you feel afraid? If so, take a deep breath and close your eyes. Focus on yourself.

Why all of this about yourself and how you're feeling when the topic is stop hurting yourself? It's simple. The biggest way that emotional eaters cause harm to themselves is by denying their own feelings and needs. Most of us were conditioned to put other people first. Combine this with the fact that we have been using food to deny our feelings and it's clear that we have little experience truly connecting with ourselves.

The next step in this process is to let others know how you are feeling once you have figured it out. This will take time and practice but once you are able to express your feelings you will find less and less need to turn to food. You will instead learn to reach out for other people. Begin by saying, "I feel _____ (fill in the blank)" out loud to someone near you.

As you go through your day today, begin to notice all of the ways you are harming yourself. Understand that the biggest way you do this is by ignoring your needs and your feelings. Begin to notice what you are feeling and what you want. You may have to stop and get silent in order to do this but that's okay. You are worth the time it takes to figure out what you are feeling and to stop hurting yourself.

65

The rewards matter more than the difficulties.

I don't think I can do this for another minute.

*I'm tired of doing all of these stupid exercises and I don't want to
read one more word about emotional eating.*

I have better things to do with my time.

ARE THESE SOME of your thoughts? Do you feel overwhelmed by all of the activities and awareness you are
experiencing? Do you feel like giving up? And, most of
all, are you feeling guilty for your thoughts?

These thoughts and feelings are normal for someone
who is undergoing any type of transition, be it a complete
lifestyle change or the ending of a small habit. When work
of any kind is required, it's easy to get discouraged. There
is no shame in feeling like quitting. This is to be expected.
Thinking about giving up is quite different from actually
going through with it.

If you try to deny your feelings you will most likely end up using food to deal with them. Instead, admit what's going on. Think about what you are feeling. Write it down if you need to. Talk about it with a trusted friend if it will help. Do whatever it takes to bring your feelings out in the open.

Then, when you feel ready, allow yourself to think about the benefits you are experiencing from this program. Have you noticed that you reach for food less often when you are upset? Are you more aware of and better able to express your feelings? Do you feel less shame about your eating habits? Have you actually cleaned out your closet and treated yourself to a reward? Are you feeling better about your life?

Even if you've only read a few entries in this book, you have still made progress by giving yourself new awarenesses. Chances are that you've done a whole lot more than that by this time. Either way, today make a list of the things you've learned and the changes you've seen in your life so far.

Refer to the list whenever you feel like giving up but don't use it as a way to deny your feelings. Simply let it serve as a reminder of all the wonderful things you are welcoming into your life through your hard work—the rewards will be obvious.

66

Inspiration may be corny, but it works.

Don't quit no matter what.
Time heals all wounds.
Quitters never win and winners never quit.
If you can dream it, you can do it.

SAYINGS SUCH AS these may be corny but they can make the difference between giving up and moving forward. A scrapbook filled with as many inspirational sayings as you can find will help. Throughout this program, you have been asked to make lists and put them in prominent places to serve as reminders. The scrapbook takes this idea a step further.

With a scrapbook, you will be able to collect as many sayings as you can. You are not limited by the size of your refrigerator or bathroom mirror. Instead, you can rip out, copy down, or paste an endless number of sayings to keep you motivated.

How you set up your scrapbook is an individual decision. You may choose to purchase a traditional book from a craft store or instead opt for a loose-leaf binder. You may want to use a small journal or even a photo album. Anything that allows you to paste, staple, or write inspirational sayings will work.

A word of caution here: It is not a good idea to simply throw bits and pieces of papers into a box or drawer. The problem with this is that you won't have easy access to looking at all of them or finding a particular saying easily. The disorganization of this system will prevent you from using it to its fullest.

Today, think about those sayings that have inspired you. Look in magazines, online, or simply write them down on a piece of paper. Then, go to the store to purchase a book to put them in or use a photo album or journal you have around the house.

Though this is an ongoing project, you can begin right now. Then, when things seem bleakest you will have a collection of inspiration right at your fingertips and one less excuse to overeat.

67

Pretending to join the Army will save your life.

REMEMBER THE OLD Army slogan, "Be all that you can be"? What does that really mean? If you were the person you've always dreamed about being, what would be different in your life today? I don't doubt that your first answer involves the size of your body and probably has all of your life. But, now it's time to look beyond that.

For many of us, our body size has been the sole focus of our lives. We have put so much time and energy into losing weight or trying to look good that we haven't paid much attention to the rest of our lives.

Right now, take a second to think about the goals you had five or ten years ago. Have they materialized? Is your life the way you hoped it would be? Did you even have goals other than those involving weight loss? Was there anything you wanted to accomplish that didn't involve your body size? If so, have you?

The point to all of this isn't to make you feel badly. Instead, it is to help you realize that there are other things in your life besides your eating habits. This isn't to say that overcoming your unhealthy patterns isn't the single most important thing in your life. It's to point out that there are other areas of your life that you may have neglected.

Unfortunately, for most emotional eaters and food addicts, life has been filled with so many failed attempts at dieting that soon this becomes the sole focus. Today, you can make a decision to take some time to get to know yourself and what you want and need in your life.

Begin to think about the things you would like to bring into your life. Have you always wanted to collect coins, travel to a foreign country, or learn to ice skate? Is painting, knitting, or pottery your passion? Would you like to work with children or be outdoors? Have you always dreamed about going back to school or switching careers?

Now, is the time to think about your life, a life that doesn't involve focusing on the size of your body. Putting some time into thinking about your future and your goals will help make room in your life for other things besides eating. This basic training will help you lead a more satisfying life—one that's focused on your goals and accomplishments, *not* on food.

68

*Standing up straight and holding your head
high will make you feel confident.*

ARE YOU HUNCHED over as you're reading this? Do
your shoulders curve forward? Is your head looking down?
What about when you walk? Do you constantly look toward
the ground?

It may seem like a simple thing to stand up straight and
hold your head high but it is not. Carrying yourself in a
confident fashion completely changes your emotional
state. Right now, sit up straight. Push your shoulders
back. Hold your head up high. Take a deep breath and look
around at your surroundings. Do you feel a difference in
the way you feel?

For some people, holding their bodies in an erect position brings on feelings of confidence while for others it is
a way to remind themselves that they are worthy. Most of us
have spent years trying to hide ourselves so that others
wouldn't pay attention to our bodies. We thought that if we
could just curl up into a little ball, no one would notice us.
And underneath it all, we felt deeply, deeply ashamed.

Today is the day that you stop allowing your shame to dictate the way you carry yourself. Instead, allow your actions to help you feel better about your body. Do this by making a conscious effort to hold your head up high and to stand up straight on a regular basis. If you are consistent and diligent about doing this, you will begin to feel better about yourself.

For many years, you have tried to think yourself into feeling better. You have done this by telling yourself that you should feel better or that you should be able to control your emotional eating. What you may have failed to realize is that rather than spending your time thinking you need to instead take action.

Today, you can make a decision to take action to feel better about your body. From this day forward, you can stand up straight and hold your head high with confidence. You are no slouch; you are worthy of feeling good about yourself.

69

You don't need to impersonate the Invisible Man.

All of their eyes were on my body. While I was covered by a loose flowery shirt and tight jeans, I was sure the only thing they could see were my layers of fat. As quickly as I could move my 328-pound body, I headed right for the farthest corner from the entrance. I knew that if I positioned myself as far away as possible, I was less likely to be noticed.

The only way I would make it through the evening would be to find a kind person who would take pity on me. She would have to be someone who wouldn't talk too loudly or dress in bold colors. My heart was pounding as I searched desperately for her. As each minute passed my heart beat stronger and stronger. I was sure it would come through my chest. Where was she? Why wasn't she here? I could see a few people beginning to look my way. I looked at the floor failing to meet their gaze. Just then, I saw her. She was petite, thin, yet plain and she had just walked through the door. She, too, was looking at the ground. Very slowly, so as not to draw attention to myself, I made my way over to her. She told me that her name was Sarah and we began to talk about the weather.

After an hour or two, when I was sure no one was looking I qui-etly slipped out the door and back to the safety of my house where I could eat everything I didn't dare at the party.

DOES ANY OF this seem familiar to you? Have you spent much of your life trying to hide in a crowd? Trying to remain invisible so no one would notice the size of your body? Or, sometimes even choosing to skip certain events that you may have enjoyed if you didn't feel so ashamed?

Today is the day to change this. Instead of hiding in a crowd stand up straight and put yourself right in the mid-dle of the festivities. Does the very thought make you shudder? Are your hands shaking as you consider the possibilities? Yet, is there a touch of excitement to think that you no longer have to feel so ashamed? That you might be able to truly enjoy yourself at a party?

Yes, you can. No matter what your body size, you have as much right to enjoy yourself and have fun as every other person in that room, including the ones who you think look perfect. By hiding yourself in a crowd, you are contributing to your feelings of shame. By allowing your-self to embrace fun, you are generating good feelings instead.

Start small. Begin with a group of three or four peo-ple in an informal situation. Go up to the group, smile, and say hello. You may want to begin by asking a question or commenting on something that happened in the news recently. You may want to practice this at work, school, the mall, the park, or anywhere else where you find yourself.

If it doesn't go as well as you hoped then try again on another day. Whatever you do, don't give up. Keep talking to every person you meet and soon you'll feel comfortable. Believe it or not, you won't have to make yourself disappear at the next party you attend.

70

Pleasing people by eating something is about you, not them.

███

Many times we tell ourselves the fat lies that we don't want to hurt someone by refusing to eat the food they have prepared. We may even let ourselves believe that we will lose friends and family members if we don't indulge.

The truth here is that eating something you feel obligated to is an indication of your need to please people and a way of further increasing your denial. The two of these work together to give you a rock solid reason to continue eating.

The thinking goes like this: If I say no to her she won't like me so I have to eat it. You convince yourself that your friendship is based solely on pleasing your friend.

While someone may be hurt if you don't eat what they have prepared, this doesn't mean the end of the relationship. Emotional eaters have difficulty realizing that other people can have feelings of anger or hurt about our actions and still remain in a relationship with us.

The feelings someone else has about you saying no are not nearly as strong or catastrophic as you might imagine.

In most cases, the person will simply hear and accept your refusal. In some, you may be urged to eat the food anyway. Understand that if you are put in the position of having to refuse food more than a few times, you may need to leave.

The single most important thing you will need to do as you continue on in this program is to put yourself first. This may sound selfish but realize that not putting yourself first is yet another way for you to create an excuse to eat. If everyone else is so much more important than you are, why shouldn't you eat?

Today is the day to change this. You are important and you deserve to feel good and healthy about your eating habits. Pleasing other people is not your job. Taking care of yourself is.

71

*Not acknowledging your beauty each day
is an ugly thing.*

THIS IS THE day that you make a decision to completely change the way you look at yourself and your body. You are no longer allowed to criticize yourself. Throughout this program, you have been asked to stop hurting yourself. Now, it is time to take this a step further.

Today, you will need to find something beautiful about yourself and continue to do so for the next nineteen days. Do you have nice hair? Are your eyes gorgeous? Do you like your hands or wrists? How about your lips or your nose? Your chest? Your legs? Your arms? What about your neck or shoulders? Are your feet attractive? Your toes or ankles? Do you have an amazing belly button or are your abs in great shape?

Your first reaction may be that you don't like any of these things. But, it's important to understand that as an emotional eater or food addict, you've trained yourself to find fault with your body. This has been going on for years. Many times it was one of the reasons you turned to food. You wanted to dull the pain of the negative feelings you have for your body. In order to change this, you will need to begin looking at yourself in a different way.

Right now, put this book down and go look in the mirror. Rather than a quick look to check your hair, look deeply into your eyes. Can you see beauty in them? Look at the color. Is there a spark there? Notice your eyelids and eyebrows. Then, really look at your nose, your chin, and your entire face. You've probably spent a lifetime finding things wrong with your face. This time, find at least two things you like.

Then continue down to the rest of your body. Observe your neck, shoulders, arms, hands, waist, hips, legs, knees, and feet. Find at least four more things about your body that are beautiful.

You may feel uncomfortable but that's to be expected. You are doing something different. Anything new, even those things that are positive, can be difficult in the beginning. For the remaining nineteen days of this program, find at least one thing that's beautiful about yourself every day.

You may want to write it down in your daily planner or in your notebook. This way you can go back and reread the entire list when you feel discouraged. Today is the day that you will begin to see yourself as the truly beautiful human being you are.

72

Magic wands don't work.

THE FIRST TIME I saw her, I hated her. Her name was Lisa and she had something I wanted. She had lost almost 200 pounds. She was smiling and happy in a way that I didn't know was possible. And she held a magic wand.

Looking me directly in the eyes she said, "I know you want me to wave this magic wand and have you lose all your weight but it doesn't work that way. You have to work for it."

The anger welled up inside of me. I didn't want to work. I wanted someone else to do this for me. And I certainly had no desire to hear what this woman was saying. My first reaction was to run as far away from her as I could. Yet, something stopped me. It was the look in her eyes. The way her face lit up. I knew instinctively that she was genuinely happy, something I had never known.

Even more surprising was the fact that she wasn't thin. After losing 200 pounds, she still weighed nearly 300 pounds—a fact she proudly told me the first day I met her. She was still overweight yet she acted as happy as if she were thin. She was like an alien to me. I never knew anyone like her existed.

Over eighteen years later, I now know the secret to Lisa's genuine happiness. She truly understood on a deep level that there are no magic wands or shortcuts to achieving peace with food. Lisa knew that having sanity in her life depended on hard work. She knew that no one else could give her what she most wanted in the world—and she became willing to give it to herself.

Today, it is my hope that you are willing to give it to yourself. It's time to take an inventory of your progress so far. Have you been doing the activities on a daily basis? Are you taking the suggestions and incorporating them into your life? Or, are you waiting for someone else to make it better for you? Are you out searching for a magic wand?

As you ask yourself these questions, think about the choices you have made over the past seventy days. Have they been ones that will lead you to where you want to go or are you falling back into the same old patterns? What kind of results are you experiencing?

Whatever answers you come up with, do not use them to beat yourself up. Instead, learn from them. If you have been lax about certain things, take action. If you don't like what's happening in your life, reach out to someone who can offer guidance while understanding that they can't save you. It is your job and your responsibility to make your life better. It will take hard work but understand that it will be worth it. Just ask Lisa.

73

Writing is the right thing to do.

████

Have you tried it yet? Did you dare to even consider going through with it? Or, have you been afraid of what you'd find?

For many of us, writing is torture. We have flashbacks of high school English classes and red marks on our papers. We tell ourselves that our grammar isn't good enough or that we can't write good sentences. Fear wells up inside of us as we think about sitting down with pen and paper.

Sometimes sitting down with a pencil and my journal is one of the most frightening things that I do during the day. In those pages I must be honest in a way that doesn't come naturally to me. I must look inside at my deepest feelings, the ones I hide even from myself, then put them down on paper and bring them into my conscious awareness.

Is it any wonder that writing is a scary prospect? Despite how frightening it may be, writing is one of the few guaranteed ways to help you overcome your emotional eating. Much of your eating happens because you unconsciously are trying to ignore your feelings. If you can learn to acknowledge your feelings, there will be less of a need to use food to hide.

Though talking to a trusted friend or family member is helpful and often nurtures us, there is no substitute for writing. Writing is a solitary process that allows you to explore your feelings in a way that talking with someone else doesn't. In other words, there's no shortcut.

It's time. Today, pick up the pen or pencil, turn on the computer, and begin to write. You don't have to write full sentences. It doesn't even have to make sense. Just simply begin to write about what you are thinking and feeling. Don't judge it. Just let it flow. When you are finished, you will know more about yourself than you did before. Now, make a commitment to write at least two times a week. Even if it's only a paragraph, just simply write. And, understand that it is truly the right thing to do if you want to overcome your emotional eating.

74

Saying no is an essential part of your healing.

W E ALL HATE to do it. There's no fun involved and we feel terribly guilty. Most times we avoid it. The problem is that to fully overcome your emotional eating, you will need to learn how to say no.

Saying no is an important part of not only your recovery but your life as well. As emotional eaters and food addicts, we often feel we have to please people to make them want to be with us. While we do this in many ways, the most common is agreeing to things we really don't want to.

Think about how many times you have said yes to helping someone when you really didn't want to. Consider how much energy you have put into doing things for others that they are capable of handling themselves. Each time you have said yes when you didn't want to, you have harmed yourself.

Sometimes this harm is small. You may not have time to take the long hot bath that you really wanted to. Other times the damage is more serious. You have given away your entire day and by the time you get home you are so angry that you binge for hours because it's the only way you know how to deal with feelings as intense as these. Either way, there is danger to yourself if you continually agree to things that you don't like or want to do.

If you're like many of us, you tell yourself that it's not so bad or that you can handle doing things that you don't want to. But, have you ever considered the price you pay by putting your desires aside to make others happy?

Chances are that you feel angry and resentful when you squash your needs. As an emotional eater, you may not recognize the way you are feeling. If you do, you may not know how to handle your emotions. Some of them may seem overwhelming. You may even try to pretend that they don't exist. Perhaps you've been raised to put on a happy face and pretend that feelings of anger and resentment don't exist.

To deal with this, you will need to learn how to say no. Today and for the rest of this program, make a decision to say no at least once a day. Start small and with someone you don't know well. If you're in the mall, for example, and someone asks you to sample a new perfume or cologne simply look them in the eye and say no. Don't offer an excuse. Just say no. Practice this for a few days then work up to saying no to family and friends.

Realize that you may feel guilty. Though it may be uncomfortable you won't die. Talk to a friend. Write about it. Take a walk. Do whatever you need to do to work through these feelings, except, of course, reach for food. You can do this. Today, start saying yes to the idea of saying no.

75

Commercials will cause cravings.

IT WAS THE first time in forty-two days and I was excited. I couldn't wait. It had been so long. My memories were sweet and I wanted to repeat the experience. After everything I had been through, I really needed an escape.

For most of my life, television had served as the ultimate distraction from the pain of my real life. Beginning in high school through college I religiously watched four soap operas daily. I spent hours thinking about the characters' lives. It was much nicer than admitting the pain of my own. Of course, as I watched, I ate the entire time. I believed this was my only escape.

Now, after returning from a six-week stay at a food addiction treatment center I was eager to once again turn on the television. Though I could no longer lose myself in four daily soap operas, I was still hopeful that escape was possible. Positioning myself on the sofa in front of the television, I felt anxious and uncomfortable. What had once seemed so familiar was now foreign.

As I flipped through the channels, I realized something was missing. Settling on a program, I tried to concentrate and managed to do so until the commercial. On the screen in full color there was a thick, juicy quarter-pound hamburger dripping with cheese and mayonnaise. How much I wanted one.

I quickly changed the channel. With forty-two days of recovery, I was not willing to lose the good feelings I had. Yet, the image of the burger seemed permanently carved in my mind. It was at that moment I knew I had never watched television without eating, even as a small child. At twenty-three years old, I had to relearn how to do something so simple. Since then, I have come to realize that the best way for me to watch television is to change the channel during commercials.

Since most advertisements are designed to play on your emotions, watching commercials is a dangerous practice for emotional eaters and food addicts. Take a second to think about some of the food advertisements you have seen throughout your life. Most times baked items are associated with giving love to your spouse or family. Sometimes, food is associated with feelings of fun, relaxation, or freedom. Either way, all of these are dangerous to your recovery.

Today, if you watch television, change the channel when the commercials come on. You don't need to be sucked back into the idea that food and emotions are tied together. You have worked too hard. You don't need to sabotage yourself by watching commercials designed to work against everything you have accomplished.

76

Baking is not the only way to show love.

"BAKE FOR SOMEONE you love." This vintage advertising slogan says it all. Baking things for someone has traditionally been considered a way to show affection. Think about the many messages we are sent on a daily basis about emotions and baked items.

In many preschools baking brownies is a regular part of the curriculum to promote teamwork and increase math skills. Children bake cookies at home and in school for recreation. In television shows, mothers bake special treats for their families to show how much they care.

These are only a few examples of the way our society has taught us that baking for others is a means of showing love. Yet, how true is this really? When you put effort into baking things for others what are you really accomplishing?

Eating foods high in fat and calories is destructive to the health of those people you love. These types of foods contribute to many health problems that actually cause harm. Obesity, heart disease, diabetes, and high blood pressure are only a few of the physical ailments that come from overeating baked goods. Emotionally, the dangers are just as serious. When we associate cookies and cake with affection we detach ourselves from truly learning how to express and receive love.

Today, make a decision to stop using baked items to express your feelings for others. Instead, learn to show love in other ways. Do something nice for those you care about that doesn't involve food. Take out the garbage. Sweep out the garage. Do the laundry. Make a special trip to the store or out to a movie. Take a drive, or attend a concert. Realize that a handmade gift or card speaks just as loud as brownies, but contains none of the unhealthy aspects. Learn to show love in new and different ways that don't involve food. You're not the only one who will be healthier for it.

77

Calories don't count.

*If I save up all of my allotted calories for the day, I can have an
entire apple pie at night. Or, if I'm really creative, I can combine
two days' worth of calorie allowances and add half a gallon of ice
cream to the pie.*

Does this sound familiar? How many times have you
done this or something similar? And when you did, what
happened? Were you successful in your healthy eating
efforts or did you continue to eat other things besides
those that fit into your daily calorie allotment?

Many of us have been trained to look at counting calories as the only means of losing weight and eating healthfully. The problem with this idea is that it deeply affects
our emotional state in a negative way. The numbers begin
to rule our lives. We feel resentful and angry about having to compute every calorie that goes into our bodies.

Similar to the way the numbers on the scale begin to
determine our emotional state, the calories in our food

become our emotional measure of the worth of the food we eat. Today is the day to change this.

Though it is necessary for food addicts and emotional eaters to have some form of portion control, counting calories simply does not work. Instead, choose a plan that allows you to weigh and measure your food. This is a more effective way to separate your emotions from food. Your plans should include a specific outline of the amounts you eat at each meal so that you cannot save everything up for one meal. Even though weighing and measuring may seem complicated, understand that it is actually easier since you will be sure to get all of the food you are entitled to.

Weighing and measuring will allow you to control your portions but will take away the obsession of calculating every bite. Your focus is broader thus allowing for less emotional attachment to your food. If this doesn't feel right for you then you may want to use plates and bowls as a means of portioning out your food. Simply use the same plate every time you eat and portion your food out into sections.

By doing this, you may find that you've enjoyed your first guilt-free meal in years, or perhaps your entire life. Use this experience to build on and make a commitment to yourself to never count calories again.

78

Food funerals help you to mourn.

LOUD SOBS FILLED the air. A large black blanket was positioned directly in the center of the circle. Women and men of various shapes, sizes, and ages stood looking down at the blanket. Most had tears on their cheeks. Some were crying uncontrollably. There was not one smile in the room of thirty-two people.

One by one each person left the circle to approach the blanket. Guided by a thin, tall, dark-haired man each one placed a piece of paper underneath the blanket. Doing so made them sob harder. One slightly plump older woman fell to her knees as she placed her paper under the blanket. The man stood nearby watching yet never reaching out to comfort her.

My heart pounded as my turn grew closer. I clutched a thin piece of paper in my right hand as I approached the blanket. On the paper were cut out pictures of potato chips, popcorn, chocolate, bread, hamburgers, and candy.

A few days before, each one of us was ordered to make collages of our binge foods using magazine photos.

Now, as I approached the blanket, I understood the full meaning of the assignment. Here before me was the blanket where I would forever place those foods that had nearly destroyed me. This was a funeral and never again would I be able to enjoy my binge foods.

As I lifted up the blanket, tears streamed down my cheeks. I fell on the floor. My hands shook as I placed the collage underneath the blanket. Barely able to breathe, I cried deeper and longer than I ever had before in my life. This was the end. I was losing my best friend forever.

Even if I did choose to eat these foods again, it would never be the same. The escape that I had once enjoyed was ruined forever by the knowledge I had gained. I could no longer convince myself that eating just one wouldn't hurt me. I knew better now. My romance with food was over forever.

As strange as this may seem, the whole process of holding a food funeral is very moving and cathartic. At first you may be tempted to judge the sanity of it all but try to put that aside and consider instead the symbolism of actually burying your binge foods. The power of this is in the act itself. It doesn't matter whether you have a room full of people or simply yourself. What's important is that you give yourself closure.

Today, grab some magazines but be careful not to let yourself get caught up in the food pictures. Instead, make a collage then find a way to bury your binge foods. You may do this by physically digging a hole in your backyard, by burning the collage, or by tearing it up into small pieces and throwing it away. Begin immediately to prepare for your food funeral. Though you may not believe that it will help, ask yourself what you've got to lose. A lifelong habit that makes you feel degraded and humiliated? Remember by deciding to bury your binge foods, you will cause the death of your emotional eating.

79

Guilt doesn't hurt as much as resentment.

"WOULD YOU BE able to help me clean out the garage on Saturday?" My friend Sue's words hung in the air between us.

My week had been overwhelmingly busy and I was very much looking forward to some rest over the weekend. Yet, Sue was one of my best friends, someone who had been there to help me when I needed it. How could I refuse?

I was torn between the guilt of wanting to say no and the resentment of actually going through with giving away my entire Saturday. I felt loyalty to Sue and was afraid that she would get angry if I didn't reciprocate the favors she had done for me.

Making decisions is one of the most challenging things for emotional eaters. Since most of us have spent a lifetime denying our needs and feelings, we have little experience in this area.

So, how do you handle this? To begin, realize that you don't have to give anyone an answer immediately. You can simply say that you'll check your schedule and get back to your friend. This will give you some time to think about the best course of action. Most times, making rash decisions is not a good idea.

The next step is to take some time to consider your options. What do you really want? At first you may be tempted to tell yourself what you think you "should" do, but try to avoid this. Be honest. Would you really prefer to refuse the request or is it no big deal for you to do it? You may want to make a list of the pros and cons about both decisions to get clearer on your thoughts. After this, take the action that supports what you truly want.

In my case, I needed to say no. Even though Sue's friendship is important to me, I understood exactly how much I needed some rest. The truth is that whatever choice I made would involve experiencing strong feelings. If I said yes then I would resent Sue and the fact that I had given up my much-needed day of rest. If I said no, I would feel guilty about being a lousy friend.

The truth is that even though I would feel guilty about saying no, that would disappear more easily than the resentment of giving up my entire day. Even though it is possible that guilt may trigger you to eat, there is no question that you will reach for food due to resentment. Resentment grows over time and gets bigger while guilt leaves you much quicker and is easier to manage. If you are paying attention to your emotions and following the program, you will be less likely to eat due to feelings that aren't as strong. Powerful feelings can be so overwhelming that eating seems to be your only option. It is always best to choose the less powerful option if you can. If you're still confused about guilt and your feelings reread entries 48, 52, and 70 to remind you.

If I had actually gone through with cleaning the garage then I would expect my friend to reciprocate not only for the chore but for the fact that I gave up my much-needed day. Chances are that this would happen on a subconscious level that I wouldn't be aware of. Any failure to more than pay back my efforts would be seen as another injustice in my eyes. Eventually, all of these so-called injustices would add up to an even bigger resentment that could result in powerful feelings and ultimately cause me to seek solace in food.

Today, if you are given the choice, choose the guilt of saying no rather than the resentment of doing something you don't want to. You will notice a difference in the way you feel.

80

Enjoying what you eat is not the same as eating everything you enjoy.

I POKED MY fork at the dry lettuce. No dressing. No croutons and no cheese. Eating this would be torture. My only other option was an equally dry bunless hamburger. No mayonnaise. No ketchup. And again, no cheese. How would I be able to stick to this way of eating for any length of time?

I couldn't. Within a matter of minutes I was in the refrigerator and shoving pieces of pizza in my mouth. I needed to eat something I enjoyed. I couldn't take the bland, dryness of the lettuce and hamburger. Bite after bite, I ate until all five pieces were gone. After that, I opened the freezer and reached for a half gallon of chocolate chip ice cream. After finishing that, I went on to eat a bag of potato chips and some cookies, leaving myself feeling nauseous and humiliated.

Today, my eating experience is completely different. I truly enjoy the food I eat. And best of all, when I sit down to a meal I know that what I am eating is healthy and I do not experience any guilt whatsoever. This is truly a miracle. Some of the foods that I eat today include: chili, scrambled eggs, sautéed vegetables, fruit mixed with yogurt, turkey loaf, rice, baked potatoes, oatmeal, and grilled eggplant.

Of course, there are many foods I enjoy that I choose not to eat today but, because I am satisfied with the things that I do have, I rarely feel deprived. Instead, unlike any of the diets I had tried before, I feel full when I've finished a meal. I no longer physically crave food nor do I feel driven to eat everything in sight.

Now, it's your turn. Today, make a decision to eat nutritious food that you enjoy but also understand that eating everything you enjoy isn't possible. Begin right now by planning a healthy meal that fits within the guidelines of your chosen food plan. Rather than eating a dry hamburger and plain lettuce decide instead to add some spice to the meat or find a healthy, lowfat dressing and add some other vegetables to that salad. Spices are a healthy way to add flavor to your food. Be careful, however, not to use too much salt. Find a way to make the food you eat appealing and you will enjoy what you eat.

81

A SWAT team will rescue you.

THEY HAVE SPECIAL weapons and are trained to assist in the gravest of emergencies. They go in when most other law enforcement officers do not. But, most of all they have special training that allows them to perform extraordinary rescues under extremely dangerous conditions.

Today, it's time to create your own SWAT team. Your battle with food is no less dangerous than the events law enforcement teams face. Though emotional eating or food addiction may not appear to be as life-threatening, it actually is. In most cases, the resolution of the crime will come quickly compared to the amount of time emotional eaters will spend suffering throughout their lifetimes if they fail to deal with their issues.

In truth, food addiction can be slow and torturous. It may take years to get help. In many cases those suffering from emotional eating never realize or deal with their issues and spend decades as victims of something they don't understand unless they reach out for help.

You have a choice. You can either be a victim or you can seek help. To do this, you need to create a support team. Similar to the SWAT teams of the early years, your own should include a minimum of four people. The reason for this is simple. No one can be available to you twenty-four hours a day seven days a week. But there will be times when you need to speak with another person. By having four people you can call in emergencies, you will guarantee yourself the help you need.

If you decide to have a smaller team, you are setting yourself up to overeat. The thinking works like this: *If my friend isn't there then I am alone and I can eat.* You will use this as an excuse to give yourself permission to overeat. Don't let yourself fall into that trap. Instead, today begin to put together your SWAT team. It can and will save your life.

82

Models may look good in print, but they don't look that good in reality.

YOU ALREADY READ that real women come in all shapes and sizes and that models and actresses exercise too much and eat too little. Consider this your final reminder about unrealistic body images. The aim of this program over the past eighty-one days has been to help you detach your emotions from food. The main way to accomplish this is by breaking down your denial mechanism—the one that tells you that you don't really have a problem or that it's not so bad. A large part of denial for emotional eaters and food addicts involves body image.

At 328 pounds, I truly believed that if I didn't tell other people I was overweight then they didn't know. Even as I write these words I find it almost impossible to believe that I actually thought this was true. Yet, it wasn't until I began working my recovery program that I understood how truly insane this belief was. Even more, I realized that believing this kept me from having to really take action. I reasoned that if no one else could see exactly how overweight I was then what did it matter?

On the other hand, I knew down to the pound what I weighed and I was all too well aware of how truly miserable I was. Whenever I saw pictures of models, the pain was even more intense. I looked at the thin figures and told myself how weak-willed and pathetic I was. Then, I headed for the kitchen to eat. If I could never look that good then I may as well eat. What I didn't realize was that each bite that I took contributed to the very problem I most didn't want.

Have you ever used photos of thin models to justify overeating? If so, it's time to understand that even models don't look that good. Remember how you read about digitally altering photographs? It's the same thing here. In these photos, body parts are made thinner, under-eye circles disappear, and abs are defined more. For the rest of us, living in reality means that we cannot magically make our bodies perfect.

Today, make a decision to stop comparing yourself to other people's bodies. Stop looking at photos of models as a means to rationalize your emotional eating. Instead, take one action today that will further your recovery program. Determine what this is by thinking about what is most troubling to you at this minute. For instance, if you are feeling lethargic because you overate last night then plan out your food for the day. Include only nutritious items. Or, if you're having trouble saying no to dangerous foods or dealing with free food then reread those entries and complete the activities outlined there. That means, actually doing what is suggested without making excuses.

Understand that the healthy truth here is that you are comparable to no one—not even those who are paid to make you believe otherwise.

83

You can't have your cake and lose weight, too.

IT'S MY BIGGEST fantasy ever, even more than winning the lottery. The one I've wanted since I was a child: being able to eat cake and lose weight too. At my heaviest, I used to shove large chunks of cake into my mouth all the while wanting to be thin more than anything else in the world. And I didn't understand why I couldn't have that.

My denial didn't allow me to understand that if I wanted to be thin, I needed to do the work involved. I had to stop eating cake and other high calorie foods. I needed to exercise and as someone who is physically addicted to foods with processed sugar and flour in them, it was imperative that I stop eating these items as well. No matter how much I may have wanted things to be different, the reality was that I couldn't eat cake and lose weight. It was not possible for me.

I had two choices. I could either continue trying to have my cake and lose weight, too, or I could accept the fact that this wasn't possible and find a way to get what I wanted.

There was no in between. I couldn't bargain my way out of the situation no matter how much I may have wanted to. The truth was that cake couldn't be a part of my healthy eating plan. It was that simple.

What about you? Whether or not you have a physical addiction to certain foods, you will still need to be completely honest about your own situation. Maybe it's not cake that's your biggest problem but whatever it is, you will need to get honest.

If you haven't already done so by this time, it's vital that you become aware of those foods that are harmful to you. Write down everything that you eat for at least a day. Do so immediately if you haven't ever before. If you did, take out the list and look at it. You need to become aware of what you're actually eating so that you can begin to make changes.

Be realistic. That's the true secret to overcoming your emotional eating and food addiction. If you can be honest about what you are eating, how it affects you, and what you need to do to change things then you will be able to have the life you've always dreamed about. And, in time, you will find as I have that there is no amount of cake that will take the place of the wonderful feelings that come from eating nutritious foods and following a recovery program.

84

Just like Linus, you will need a blanket.

Y OU'VE SEEN HIM for years dragging his blanket wherever he goes. Sometimes he holds it closely. Other times
it sits on the floor right next to him. Either way, the blanket is always there. Famed cartoonist Charles M. Schulz
knew a thing or two about providing security for his characters when he created Linus and gave him a blanket.
Now, it's your turn.

No matter how diligent you are about working through
this program, there will come a time either during these
ninety days or afterward that you will be tempted to stray.
That's the reality of following a healthy eating plan in a
world that is designed to encourage overindulgence.
Today, you have a chance to prepare for that moment.

Now that you've worked through most of the activities
in this book you have more knowledge about yourself and
your feelings than ever before. You are aware of some of
the emotions that trigger you to reach for food. You've
shed some light on the sneaky ways you use food and

you've even looked at the messages you send yourself about your body. All in all you've done a great deal of work that has resulted in greater self-knowledge than ever before.

Armed with your new awareness, you can now find your own blanket to comfort you when things seem overwhelming. I'm not suggesting that you carry a blanket with you wherever you go. Instead, find an object to carry with you that reminds you of your commitment to your new way of life. It can be anything from a coin with a special saying on it, a piece of jewelry, a special stone, a religious object, or an inspirational passage.

The day my own object came, my hands shook as I slowly opened the black velvet box. I knew that this was a very special piece of jewelry. All special jewelry comes in fancy boxes. Flipping the lid up, tears filled my eyes as I looked at the large silver ring with a sapphire in the middle. On one side, my initials were carved and, on the other, the date of my first day of recovery. Around the sapphire were the words "To thine own self be true."

Falling to my knees, I said a silent prayer of thanks. This ring symbolized my commitment to a healthy way of life. It was a testament to the hard work that I had done and to that to come. It meant that no matter what happened in my life, I would not ever sacrifice my recovery program for anything else in the world. It was a true commitment to myself. I wear this ring today and when things are difficult I only need to look at my left hand to remind myself that no matter what happens I will be okay as long as I continue working my program. My ring is a constant reminder of the security I have in being true to myself and continuing to do what I have for the past eighteen years.

Today, take some time to look for something special to remind you of your commitment. Your object doesn't have to be expensive. It just has to mean something to you. So, go ahead and learn a lesson from Linus. Find your own blanket.

85

Using food in the décor of your home is like playing with a loaded gun.

██████

AREN'T THEY CUTE? Dish towels with big red apples on them. Or, how about the wallpaper boarder with a basketful of vegetables? Wouldn't that make a nice addition to the kitchen? In the dining room, there are even blown glass bananas from that trip to Bermuda.

What could possibly be wrong with using nutritious food in the décor of your home? Six words: out of sight, out of mind. It goes without saying that using high calorie foods in your décor is akin to playing with a loaded gun. Yet, most people don't realize that even food that's healthy can cause difficulties for emotional eaters and food addicts.

The point of the past eighty-four days has been to break the emotional bond you have with food. Every exercise that you've completed, every entry that you've read, and every step forward that you've taken has all been to put food in its proper place, as a means of nourishing your body not feeding your emotions.

If you've gotten all of the junk food out of your house and the only thing left to eat when you feel tempted is food on your plan, you may reach for that. Sometimes it's easier to justify overeating foods that are acceptable than those that are clearly dangerous.

Today, look around your house and remove all reminders of food in your décor. Do you have an apple paperweight? Is there a tablecloth with vegetables on it? What about the kitchen rug? Do you have one of those that has a watermelon design on it? What about the other rooms? Is there artwork with food on it? Remove it all!

And though avoiding food in the décor of your home may seem extreme when you are feeling strong, it will not be that way when you feel weak or overwhelmed. The reminders of food may cause you to reach for something that will ultimately cause harm to your body. Is that really worth it?

86

Love is all you need.

You've heard it before. The lyrics are from the famous Beatles' song *All You Need Is Love*. But what does this have to do with overcoming your emotional eating? It's actually quite simple. Once you have stopped using food to deal with your emotions and learned about your feelings, you will need to learn how to love yourself. Most of us have never been told how to love ourselves or even that it's important that we learn how.

Today is the day to think about it and also to begin. Where do you start? Put this book down. Go look in the mirror deep into your eyes. Say the words, "I love you." Go ahead. Do it right now then come back.

How did that feel? Was it the same feeling as when someone special tells you that they love you? Or, did you feel as if you wanted to burst into tears? If you didn't use a mirror, go do so now. Simply saying it to yourself without looking in the mirror isn't as effective. Like with everything else in this program, half the effort results in half the progress.

The first time I looked in the mirror into my eyes and said "I love you" I burst into tears. I sobbed for several minutes. I didn't understand what was happening but I couldn't stop the tears, either. What I realize now is that I had been so critical and mean to myself that it was painful for me to actually be nice to myself. I was deeply sad for all of the abuse I had suffered at my own hands. As time went on and I continued to do this, it got easier and eventually I began to believe it.

Now, it's your turn. For the next thirty days, look in the mirror every morning deep into your eyes and say "I love you." Even though it may feel uncomfortable at first, don't give up. Keep at it and it will get easier. You, too, will come to find that love—not food—is all you need to change the way you feel about yourself.

87

Emotional hunger isn't physical and shouldn't be treated that way.

CHOCOLATE CHIP ICE cream. It was all I could think about. The way the creaminess of it would feel against my tongue as it danced in my mouth. The thought of the crunchy chocolate chips coupled with the rich vanilla flavor would surely make everything better. How could kids be so mean? The awful things they had said to me.

"Fatso! Fatso! Fatso!" They chanted so loudly the entire school could hear. I wanted to shrivel up and die but I had been forced to continue walking in the direction of my house as they grew louder and louder following me down the driveway and around the corner. Thankfully, they had grown tired once they reached the small convenience store.

With shaking hands and tears in my eyes, I reached inside the freezer and grabbed a half gallon of ice cream. It didn't matter that I had just eaten lunch. It didn't matter that my feet ached from the short walk home. All I cared about was tasting the coolness of the ice cream. There was no stopping myself as I shoved spoonful after spoonful into my mouth, barely hesitating to even breathe, practically choking as the heaping piles of ice cream slid down my throat.

When I was finished, my stomach ached. I felt ashamed and humiliated by my lack of control, and my head was pounding. I curled up under the covers and cried myself to sleep. I wanted to be thin more than anything else in the world yet I couldn't seem to stop eating. . . .

What I experienced then was not physical hunger. You can probably see that my eating was triggered by a deep misguided need to nurture myself and eating was the only way I knew how to do that. My guess is that though your emotional eating episodes may not have been as dramatic you have still experienced something similar.

In order to end your emotional connection to food, you need to create different behaviors. This entry is about reinforcing that and taking inventory of your progress. Today, if you are still unsure what physical hunger feels like then go back through this book and reread some of the entries. If you haven't done any of the suggested activities or if you've skipped over some go back and do those. Being honest with yourself is the only chance you have at learning to separate physical hunger from emotional cravings. Your life depends on it so don't quit now!

88

Burning something will light a fire under your recovery.

BEFORE YOU GO out and burn something, read this all the way through. I don't mean go out and burn down a house or anything like that. What I am suggesting is a symbolic burning to release past pain or present anger.

Imagine that you are so angry at your best friend that you want to strangle her. Rather than screaming at her, ignoring your feelings, or turning to food to deal with them, you can try something different. First, write a letter to her explaining exactly why you are so angry. Don't hold anything back. Call her every name in the book. Get it all out on paper. You may even want to bring up anything from the past that's bothered you. Write and write until you have gotten all of it out.

Now, this is the important part. Don't even think about sending it to your best friend. Instead, go near the fireplace, the sink, or even the bathtub. Read the letter once more out loud. Yell if you need to. Then, light the match and set the letter on fire, being careful, of course, not to burn yourself. Watch the letter burn and as you do imagine all of your anger being sucked away by the flames. When most of it has burned extinguish the fire to prevent it from spreading.

After you have finished, take a few minutes to either jot down your thoughts about how you feel or to discuss your experience with a trusted friend. How did it feel to write about your anger and watch it burn? How do you feel right now? You may still be angry but what you have done is to take the intensity out of your feelings.

At some point, you may need to discuss your feelings with your friend in a calm, rational manner. The best way to do this is to use the "I feel (or felt) _____ when you _____" formula. It works like this. In a calm voice simply state your feelings about the event saying something similar to this: I felt angry when you were late for the movie. You may or may not want to elaborate on this by discussing any other feelings you had such as hurt or sadness.

Be careful, however, not to blame your friend. This is about stating your feelings. All of the things you wrote in the letter were so that you could get out the most intense feelings before discussing them with your friend. Reading the letter you wrote will most likely destroy the friendship. Stating how you feel in a healthy way will create even greater intimacy in the relationship.

After reading all of this, your first thought may be why bother? Why can't you just forget about it and move on? The reason is quite simple—if you deny your feelings and don't talk about them, you will reach for food. In order to truly overcome your emotional eating, you need to change the way you deal with your feelings. You can no longer hide them or pretend that they don't exist. You will need to acknowledge then release them. So, go ahead, light a fire under your recovery.

89

Growing pains are part of life.

Today, it is important to take a step back and give yourself credit for your awarenesses and accomplishments. If you've completed all or most of the activities during the previous eighty-eight days, you've taken some big steps forward. You've probably realized some valuable things about your behaviors and actions. Chances are that none of this has been as easy as you would have liked.

Though you can most likely recognize the value in this growth process, you may be tired. And if you haven't completed all of the activities, you may even be discouraged or frustrated with yourself. You might even be using the appearance of your lack of progress as an excuse to overeat. Before you pick up the food, continue reading.

Understanding the growth process will help you to be prepared when feelings of discouragement begin to pop up. Growing, whether it's the physical growth of a person, animal, or plant, doesn't always happen in a straight line. Sometimes in order to move two steps forward we must first take one step backward. This is normal and to be expected. Even with one step backward, you have still made one step forward.

During your recovery from emotional eating, you will face many challenges but with the things you have been learning over the past three months, you will have a good foundation to continue moving forward. You may have to rest or stop growing for a short time. It is all part of the process. The best thing you can do at this point is to remind yourself that you are making progress. The easiest way to do this is to have a physical reminder of how the growth process unfolds.

Today, buy yourself a plant or a pet or anything else that you can watch grow. As you see your plant or pet growing, constantly remind yourself of your own progress. Use this to remind yourself of your commitment to overcoming your emotional eating and as a symbol of your continued progress.

The danger you face is the temptation to stop working on your recovery. Having a physical, growing reminder of your commitment will help you to continue moving forward. So, go ahead, grow something.

90

You are worth it.

Y OU'VE WORKED HARD. You've learned a lot about yourself. You've faced some difficult challenges and yet still continued to work through them. Even if you simply read each entry without doing the activities, you have created an awareness that you can use to build on. Whatever you have done or not done, you have made progress.

Though this is the end of the first ninety days, it is important that you continue on in your journey to overcome emotional eating and food addiction. You cannot simply do this for ninety days and be cured for the rest of your life. The truth is that you will need to continue doing many of the things you have learned during these ninety days.

At this point, you may feel overwhelmed by the thought of doing these things for the rest of your life. This is to be expected. The way to deal with this is to only think about today. You don't have to live your whole life in this one day. Instead, you can think only about the next twenty-four hours in front of you. If you make this the best day possible then the rest of them will be taken care of. This is one of the most powerful tools I can pass along to you.

It's been over eighteen years since I've had a cookie or a piece of bread, ice cream, or cake. When I first began following my food plan, I didn't believe that I could do it for eighteen minutes never mind more than eighteen years. I did believe, however, after my first day on the plan that I could do it for one day. I knew that if I made a phone call when I wanted to eat or took a walk when things got too emotional that I could get through four meals that day.

Some of those days were easier than others. There were days that I simply breezed through and there were ones that seemed to last forever. But, whatever happened during those twenty-four hours, I made a decision to never, ever give up. And somehow, each day began to add up to over eighteen years. It wasn't magic. It was hard work and constant vigilance. And it was worth every single bit of effort.

Today, I no longer feel completely devastated and ashamed from overeating. I do not feel sick to my stomach and filled with self-hatred. Instead, I enjoy an incredible freedom. Most days, I do not obsess or think about food. I can walk into a store and buy clothes that fit and I can eat and enjoy my meals without guilt or shame. My life is truly a miracle.

This is what I wish for you—recovery from your emotional eating and food addiction. Please know that it is possible and that you can do it. You will need to work for it but it will be worth every bit of the effort involved. You are worth it.

RESOURCES

████

THANK YOU FOR sharing this journey with me. I truly
wish you the best. Please feel free to write to me if you have
any questions or want to share your experience: Debbie
Danowski, 4 Daniels Farm Road, 193, Trumbull, CT
06611 or debbie@debbiedanowski.com.

Here are some more resources to help you along your
journey:

ONLINE SUPPORT FOR EMOTIONAL EATERS
AND FOOD ADDICTS:

Overeaters Anonymous online meetings:
www.oa.org/online_meetings.html

Food Addicts Anonymous online meetings:
www.foodaddictsanonymous.org/online.htm

ACORN Recovery Community:
www.health.groups.yahoo.com/group/
acorncommunity/

HealthyPlace.com:
www.healthyplace.com/

Free Newsletter:
www.debbiedanowski.com

FOOD ADDICTION TREATMENT:

ACORN Food Dependency Recovery Services
P.O. Box 50126
Sarasota, FL 34232-0301
Phone: (941) 378-2122
Fax: (941) 346-0187
E-mail: ACORNInfo@foodaddiction.com
Web site: www.foodaddiction.com

Overeaters Anonymous
World Service Office
P.O. Box 44020
Rio Rancho, NM 87174-4020
Phone: (505) 891-2664
Fax: (505) 891-4320
Web site: www.oa.org/index.htm

Food Addicts Anonymous
4623 Forest Hill Blvd., Suite 109-4
West Palm Beach, FL 33415-9120
Phone: (561) 967-3871
Fax: (561) 967-9815
E-mail: info@foodaddictsanonymous.org

Turning Point of Tampa
6227 Sheldon Road
Tampa, Florida 33615
Phone: (813) 882-3003
Toll-free: (800) 397-3006
Fax: (813) 885-6974
Web site: www.tpoftampa.com

ACKNOWLEDGMENTS

I AM TRULY blessed to have many wonderful and supportive people in both my professional and personal life. Professionally, my agent Linda Konner and editor Renée Sedliar at Avalon are both equally amazing. Their dedication to making this book as successful as possible is truly a gift. In addition to this, my first editor Corrine Casanova and my mentor Dr. Ralph Corrigan continue to shape and guide my writing career.

The staff at Avalon has been wonderful. Also, my coworkers at Sacred Heart University offer me an incredible amount of support on a daily basis and I remain grateful. Though there are too many to mention, it is important that each and every one of them knows how much they mean to me.

I am also blessed with a strong community of writers in my life. My writers group with Jessica Bram, Aly Dune, Lucy Hedrick, Joanne Kabak, and Jane Pollak provided a great deal of support during the writing of this book and also in my personal life. We are far more than simply a writers group. We are friends. Other writers and friends in my life whom I am equally grateful for are Lisa Blackman, Mark Edwards, Dawn Rosner, and Cindy Simoneau. I am also grateful for magazine editors Matt Kolk of *Fairfield County Home* and Deb Owens of *Fairfield* magazine.

Additionally, the work that Phil Werdell, and ACORN Food Dependency Recovery Services and the Food Addiction Institute staff and advisory board are doing is so important in my life and in many other people's. I am grateful for all that they do and for all whom they have helped, including me.

I would also like to acknowledge each and every one of the people who have read my previous three books and taken the time to write to me. Your letters and e-mails mean so very much to me. I am grateful that you are so generous with your praise and humbled by the fact that my words have helped you to change your lives.

Personally, my parents, Andy and Ann, have offered me support my entire life. And though my mother is no longer here, she was with me as I wrote every word. I am also grateful for my sister, Karen, and brother-in-law, Danny, my brother, Mike, and sister-in-law, Denise, my niece, Melissa, and my niece, Felicia, as well as my extended family.

The past two years have been emotionally challenging and I know that I would not have made it through this without my friends who have offered me incredible support never once asking for anything in return. They are: Debby Adkinson, Amy Day, Karen Kahn Wilson, Roger Stolz, Alex Minutillo, and Beverly Robillard.

I would also like to acknowledge a group of people who have come to mean more to me than I can ever say. Those who support me on Mondays and Fridays at noon, and Mondays and Thursdays at 6:00 PM, and Saturdays at 4:00 PM have given me the very life I have today. There are no words to acknowledge the gratitude I feel for having so much support.

Finally, it would be impossible not to acknowledge two people whom I love dearly. Olivia Kashetta, though we've only just begun our relationship, is very special to me and I am grateful for her presence in my life. And, Charlie Kashetta, who means more to me than words can ever say. His love and support over the past two years have changed my life. I am truly blessed by my relationship with him. Thank you, God.